HEALTHIOLOGY 101

HEALTHIOLOGY 101

The Active Body Culure Self-Testing
Health Quiz and Game Book for
Individuals, Institutions and
Corporate Wellness

M. M. WILSON

iUniverse, Inc.
New York Lincoln Shanghai

Healthiology 101
The Active Body Culure Self-Testing Health Quiz and Game Book for
Individuals, Institutions and Corporate Wellness

iUniverse books may be ordered through booksellers or by contacting:

iUniverse
2021 Pine Lake Road, Suite 100
Lincoln, NE 68512
www.iuniverse.com
1-800-Authors (1-800-288-4677)

Because of the dynamic nature of the Internet, any Web addresses or links contained in this book may have changed since publication and may no longer be valid.

ISBN: 978-0-595-47103-4 (pbk)
ISBN: 978-0-595-91616-0 (cloth)
ISBN: 978-0-595-91385-5 (ebk)

Printed in the United States of America

This book is **not** a substitute for advice from licensed doctors or therapists. It is a book to awaken your knowledge that good health is not mere absence of disease. Regardless of medical advances and doctors, they cannot replace the individual's responsibility for every day good health practices. The game is a lifestyle changing game to help you learn more about your own body and how you can prevent certain diseases from occurring or how to maintain whatever disease you already have so you can benefit from a better quality of the life that is left in you.

Art by Gordon Szendrey
Design by iUniverse

Contents

Acknowledgment

First and foremost I would like to thank the inner spirit for inspiring me to write a book that lends a hand to people's health and wellness. This is a book which will enable us to put our health first, when we learn to take the self-testing questions, in the form of a game. Without such inner guidance I could not have written this book, looking for something so basic that could help prevent certain diseases or save lives, in each of the question posed.

Dad died in February 2004 from diabetes. I owe this to everyone I know, and the readers I will meet, in the pages of the *Healthiology* book or board game, to tell you, we can do it. I am also indebted to you, to tell you that many diseases are avoidable, and prevention is the cornerstone. We need to take care of our health into our own hands, because nobody will do it for us.

I met a new friend, Lea, who has multiple sclerosis, and her disease has helped changed my life forever. Her MS is termed chronic-progressive, making her almost impossible to take care of her basic needs. Her story has inspired me to write on common sense for *everyday* health.

I wish to offer my sincere thanks to all who helped me to deliver from the medical questions that eventually became the pages of this *Healthiology* book and board game. Without you, I would have stunted to come up with meaningful health questions, relevant for a game and book, to make it fun and learned at the same time. Thank you, all.

And, of course, what's a book without the editors and contributing editors? To Odette Hyatt, Anita Bell, Sylvia Allen and Joyce Standish who have worked on the editing of the game book for me, to you, I say thanks with much appreciation. From the first moment your eyes saw the manuscript, you believed in the importance of telling *Healthiology's* story, and your enthusiasms for this book never lagged, to tell your own family and friends that good health is not a destination, but a day-by-day journey.

I owe a special debt of gratitude to my grandchildren. Their ever-present love was even more deeply felt during the writing of this health game book. I will help them take health-ownership of their bodies, in their young lives. I want them not to get caught in someone else's shadow, but to grow in their own skin, weight and space, and enjoy their life to include visualization—a solid foundation for self-empowerment about health, happiness, dreams and aspirations.

Introduction

We are living longer than ever, but do you want to live in chronic pain, disease and misery, if you can avoid it? The *Healthiology 101* game will help you to reflect on your own health and others around you, like your children or spouse, and how to prevent some diseases from happening.

Some of us live in countries that pays for some or all our medical expenses, while others live in countries where you have to pay for your own health benefits, no matter what, which sometimes run into hundreds or even thousands of dollars each month. Whether you live in a country that pays or do not pay for your medical bills, the key is to know about preventable diseases, and how to maintain healthy lifestyles to prevent these diseases.

There is something within each of us that values how we look on the outside rather than how we look on the inside. But the inward quality is what counts, as it will reflect on the outside, which is important to good health.

Think of a newborn child like a new car. The newborn is healthy and just the way it is when you purchase that well made car. Over time and after driving the car for a number of years you will find that it needs maintenance and new parts. So it is, if you fail to give a child the proper nutrition, sooner or later that child will not have resistance to fight off flu or colds; they might even stop growing healthy and strong. They need proper nutrients in their bodies to grow up healthy and strong. A car cannot run on water and would need petrol for you to drive it everyday. The same methods apply to a child. They cannot grow without good nutrition, exercise and plenty of sleep everyday.

When you read this, remember that some diseases are heredity while others are preventable. So the one thing we all can savor is to: *Eat a well-balanced diet, exercise regularly, meditate, drink lots of water and get plenty of sleep; get regular medical check-ups—at least once a year, as part of our ongoing health lifestyle changes.* The mission of this game is to provide knowledge to people of all ages, circumstances and interests that your health should become a number one issue and not weight. It is our bad habits that are killing us. Focus on simple, but healthier habits, not only on size or weight.

The notable American, President Franklin Roosevelt, once said, "We cannot be a strong nation unless we are a healthy nation, and so, we must recruit not only men and women and material but also knowledge and science in the service of national strength." Those were the words of President Roosevelt, taken from his address at the dedication of the National Institute of Health in October 1940. His words bring new meaning to health in the twenty-first century, as we live in a time of uncertainty, which places more stress on human lives.

The only place where 'success' comes before 'work' is in the dictionary. Therefore, to gain success with your health, you must work at it. With this game, one will learn about the prevention of diseases and how to work to achieve good health. The truth is disease prevention can only be achieved when individuals know what to do to prevent them, and to take economic and health security into their own hands. My dad died in the twenty-first century from diabetic coma, an age which saw one of our most advanced stages of medicine. Though dad had a preventable disease, he died because of lack of knowledge. I believe this game can answer some of the simplest forms of prevention about people's health and well being—and help them to take control of their health.

I firmly believe that *prevention* is better than *cure*, and many diseases that are chronic, prevention is the key. Prevention is also much healthier and still cheaper than medical research and, is therefore something that everyone should embrace and practice for good health.

The *Healthiology 101* game is an exciting knowledge-based healthy game for adults to begin taking ownership of their bodies and hence pass it down to their children and the sooner they begin the process of good health care the healthier they will be as they grow up. This is the prevention stage.

Once prevention is undermined, the next step is medical research. Both prevention and medical research is the key to eliminating diseases, reducing human suffering, and thus reducing health care costs. However, *prevention* is far most effective than *medical research*. For example, heart disease and cancer, the two leading cause of death among Americans, constitute nearly one-fifth of America's health care bill.

Some diseases are not preventable, like Multiple Sclerosis (MS) or Alzheimer's disease, but the benefits to maintain good healthy lifestyles with these diseases are far more rewarding with this game. For example, Alzheimer's disease devastates 4 million Americans and currently cost $100 billion dollars each year and is expected to increase dramatically as baby boomers age. "Fighting Diseases With Checkbooks," published in *The New York Times* on Saturday, July 8, 2006 stated:

> "We exist only as long as wealthy individuals, through their philanthropies, continue to donate to the causes they support, like Michael R. Milken for prostate cancer and Michael J. Fox for Parkinson's dis-

ease, are growing forces behind medical research. But it does present a significant risk to rely on a few philanthropic organizations and government cutbacks. The World Health Organization does not have the power to get enormous amounts of things happening quickly. Of course, reliance on philanthropies, government and private individuals, does not make up for practicing good health. Government can change courses, when administrations change, and programs can be tangled in politics."

As been reported, in 2005 alone, the Michael J. Fox Foundation for Parkinson's Research is spending approximately $25 million on research. Meanwhile Fibrosis Foundation spent $100 million or Therion Biologics who raised $100 million for the development of a so-called cancer vaccine, only to announce that its pancreatic cancer treatment failed to prolong lives. These are the more reasons why everyone need to play this game.

Diseases will rape the body of its sight, hearing, mobility, and the use of many functions and can also cause people to experience low morale. The economic costs of disease—not to mention the human costs—are truly staggering. It cost companies billions of dollars each year to pick up the slack for employees who are off sick each month; some illnesses that are substantial due to lack of exercise or healthy eating.

Of course, some diseases are bound to happen, but when faced with such unavoidable disease, one needs to maintain their health to withstand the disease, not to further deteriorate their health at a speed or need to constantly live on medication. Parkinson's disease afflicts nearly a half million Americans and costs at least $6 billion a year. Nearly half a million Americans suffer strokes each year, costing more than $30 billion for medical treatment, rehabilitation, and long-term care, as well as lost wages. Diabetes, which badly affects nearly 16 million Americans, costs between $90 billion and $140 billion annually and is the leading cause of blindness and kidney disease. Although my dad was not part of the American's equation of the approximate $140 billion diabetes costs or the $250 billion spent on prescription drugs alone in 2005. (Dad was part of the Canadian health care costs whose government paid for his medical expenses, but there are many citizens of other countries who are not so lucky.) Increased poor health has deeply impacted the development of this health quiz book and board game. I want to make a difference to the health care system, and this game would bring health awareness to the world-at-large.

According to the U.S. Census Bureau's latest statistics, baby boomers, those born between the years 1946 and 1964 are 78.2 million. It is projected that more than seven hundred people turned age sixty each day in 2006. There are nearly forty-nine million Americans with disabilities and half a billion worldwide. It is estimated that there are also approximately forty-seven million Americans without medical insurance. How to stop the economic and human cost of these diseases? Prevention is the key and Research is secondary.

Many diseases can be prevented, less intrusively and with greater success if proper care and exercise is adhered to. What about children living with obesity? The increasing significant growth of children with obesity is out of control, and this sense of equality is what this game is about. And we cannot forget anorexia nervosa, as so many children and adults are living with this disease, because they are afraid of gaining weight. Anorexia nervosa is a serious, chronic and life-threatening disorder, and it too is out of control with children as young as five years old.

The *Healthiology* game was created to encourage children to grow up with a healthier mindset, and to help them take ownership of their bodies from early on in life. It is an educational and family game where children are the center of it all, and they get to see the process of living healthy verses living unhealthy by playing the game.

The truth is: In one year alone, four hundred ninety-five thousand (495,000) women in America lost their lives to cardio-vascular diseases. While, $100 billion dollars spent on Alzheimer's treatment, $30 billion for stroke victims medical treatment, rehabilitation and long-term care, between $90 and $140 billion on diabetes, and $250 billion spent on prescription drugs. How to get individuals to take responsibility of their health? Yelromusa.com has developed a board game to substitute for this book for younger children, to encourage young minds to venture into learning about healthy lifestyles that will lead them on the path of good nutrition and exercise. The board game has a human touch and interaction that can help bring awareness of good health. The players get the joy of playing a game that could become a learning route to help children, parents, hospitals, nursing colleges and homes, daycare centers, and school cafeterias become better equipped on how to choose the right nutrition and exercise that will lead them to healthier lifestyles.

Not Just Another Book

The *Healthiology 101* book is not just another book. The difference, it's a book that can improve kids or adults chance of wellness by helping them to develop better care for eating and exercise habits. There has been a lot of talk about health, but not a lot of aggressive action has been taken to let people understand that the fundamental of good personal health care only calls for a lifestyle change. We have weathered away from healthy eating, so *Healthiology* is doing less talking and has taken a more proactive role by lending a hand in a health care game book that turns fun and play into common sense action.

Good health does not come in the form of a pill; neither does health come in the form of a medical surgery procedure or treatment. With *Healthiology 101*, you will be able to learn a lot about prevention. For example, the horrible disease of osteoporosis is a lack of calcium called calcium deficiency. Such a disease is preventable or become chronic if you know what to do and how to take care of your health.

Taking care of your health has never been so easy. You can become a genius to good healthy living by playing this healthy lifestyle game. This book is not a propaganda machine to brainwash you about your health. This is a game that can get everyone more hype to taking care of their own health. If you understand your health better you are bound to take care of your health and well being.

The best medicine of protecting your health is for you to take care of yourself. Once you learn how this game is played, you'll not only have lots of fun, but also you'll be protecting yourself and family on the premise of looking after your health. For instance, healthy eating and exercise can help reduce stress, sickness and unhappiness, but too often emphasis is placed only on body image. We are more concerned about how we look from the outside instead of how we feel from the inside. Subsequently, all our goals are placed on dieting. And that is the reason why diets don't work, because we are obsessed with too thin or too fat, when really it's more than just that. Good health starts from inside-out to be effective.

Living healthy is not all about diets. For diets to work, we first have to know about our own body-type. Diets do not work from the results available to us, as we can see from the many thousands of books written about dieting and over forty-three millions Americans on diets. We also need to know that food or exercise alone does not change anything. We first have to get in touch with our inner self for food and exercise to advantageously work on our mind, body and spirit. I hope this game book will help get a mindset on the road to excellent health discovery.

From the moment we were born we become disconnected with our whole being. We are fed with unhealthy foods that contain trans fat, saturated fat, high sodium and high cholesterol levels, making us fragile to many illnesses. These foods are harmful to our bodies. At first we were not able to do anything about it, because we were babies. Then we grew up eating the same bad foods our parents gave us, did little or nothing to exercise because we did not know any better. And finally, we past down these same bad habits to our children, one generation after another. Now suddenly we want to change those lifetime bad habits in a day or two. But nothing is going to happen so quickly, because we are going about it the wrong way.

The wrong way to get and stay healthy is to want to be somebody else. We want to emulate a model—a stranger we have never met, except seen on television or in a magazine. We want our noses to look like theirs, including our cheeks, faces, breasts or stomachs. We want that person's shape or figure. What we failed to see or understand is that person we see in the magazine or on television may have spent thousands of dollars on plastic surgery or other means to look superficially good. Or perhaps, the person has good genes or is dedicated to healthier lifestyles. They ate well-balanced meals, worked out at least 30 minutes a day, drank lots of water and got plenty of sleep. And that is not all—airbrush and make-up do wonders to the face and body.

We can reverse the way we look and feel once we get to personally know our bodies. The *Healthiology* game approach is to help us find ourselves and move past the body-abuse to a joyful experience of who we really are. This book can help us to live healthier, as it is open-minded about something so important: Good health is not the mere absence of diseases. Regardless of medical advances and doctors, they cannot replace an individual's responsibility for every day good health practices.

Playing the game allows us to understand the fundamentals and dynamics of our own bodies. We have wondered away from healthy eating and playing the game helps you go back to simplicity and common sense of eating a well-balanced diet and exercise.

Eating a well-balanced meal, in this game book, means *eating from creation*. What that means is: You need to eat grains, nuts, seeds, fruits and vegetables and stop messing up your body with artificial foods. Until then, we may never get the joy of looking good and staying healthy from the inside out.

This book opens up a whole new category of the meaning of quality of health, which was long overdue. The *Healthiology* game was created in a book and board game form to help children to grow up with a healthier mindset, and to help them take ownership of their bodies from early on in life, with the help of responsible adults. It is an educational family game where children are the center of it all. The saying goes, "Practice makes improvement," and both the board game and book were developed to encourage young minds to venture into learning about good health that will eventually lead them on the path of good nutrition and exercise.

The book has a human touch and interaction that can help bring awareness of good health in both young and old. The board game adds that family touch of getting the entire family or friends to play along. We not only get the joy of playing a game, but something so pivotal that could become a learning tool to help children, parents and schools become better equipped on how to choose the right nutrition and exercise that will lead us to healthier lifestyles. You can play the game alone, just like reading a novel or science fiction, or it can be played along with other players. This way we can answer the skill testing questions, *A, B or C.*

The *Healthiology* game represents the interests and responsibilities of adults and children in order to secure their present and future health. So don't compromise. Learn this game and transform the healthy way to our children so they can develop good nutritional values. In doing so, the game opens up a dialogue and will let us become more comfortable talking about our bodies, knowing what is happening inside and outside of our bodies as well. As we take care of ourselves, becoming more and more familiar with nutritional food intake, exercise benefits, signs and symptoms of lifestyle diseases, we are definitely on our way to looking better and staying healthier.

Does Size Matters?

The problem we see is not about size as much as about someone becoming obsessive with being 'too thin' or 'too fat' in our every day life. You do not have to be a size 0 to be beautiful or a size 24 to be unattractive. You can look terrific no matter what you weigh. What you need that is more important for your existence to truly appreciate yourself living in this picturesque world is to love the body you are in. Have you ever stopped once in a while and ask yourself this question: *Am I healthy?* Unmask your health, do not treat your body like a *thing* but treat it like a *human being*, and learn to take care of the only body you will ever have by stop worrying about your size over your health.

A positive self-image is also important, but not as vital as having a good mental health. Good mental health is far more rewarding than self-image, so do not lag your health behind and put size in front. Allow your mental health to help you to shine from the inside out. The only way to do that is to practice, as practice makes improvement and not perfect as you have been led to believe, because nobody will ever be perfect.

You cannot eat nothing and still be healthy, and you cannot eat all you want and lose weight. That's only a perception. You must adhere to good diets, exercise and so forth. By practicing good healthy behaviors will give you that special edge to love yourself, take care of your body, and get to the size you so desire. A train of thought is never allow your size to clog your thoughts with negativity, because that can take away your happiness or kills your good feelings or invades your brain space, which will consent to you getting negative thoughts about the way you look or feel. Learn to grow in your own skin, weight, and space. Take care of your health by introducing nutritiously sounding diets, get regular exercise and visit your doctor to get annual medical check ups; then you may not have to worry as much about your size.

Does size matters? Size matters when it invades your brain space and clogs up your thoughts. It matters when your visualization skills allow you to create only negative mental images about *you*. Create a visualization about your health, and stop focusing on your size. When you practice good healthy habits you are bound to see positive results, as results can only be accomplished by your actions to produce positive energies and good mental health. Take care of yourself without the worry of being a size 0 or a size 24, but rather about doing what is important to look good, feel loved and staying healthy.

Remember you are the navigator who is in charge of your personal health and wellness. Only you can make that change in *your* self. Therefore, you have nobody else to blame, but yourself, if you do not take charge of your own health by practicing good health keeping.

How To Be Me

Before you begin to play the *Healthiology* game, you need to stop doing something right now. Stop being obsessed with the either 'too thin' or 'too fat' syndrome and become yourself, because you really cannot be someone else. Health is not about starvation, purging or over-eating or it's not about being thin or fat, but loving who we are and learn to maintain a healthy weight by learning to be good to our bodies and to one another.

Have you allowed magazine or television images to use their power of influence to steal your good health judgment with thin models? If so, it can be restored and maintained when you stop being weathered away from healthy eating, daily exercise and regular medical check-ups.

The foundation for health is first finding yourself and build the foundation in practical ways. Dieting is like a 'blame game'. We tend to blame others or things than ourselves for poor health choices. When we eat poorly and do not exercise enough we should take responsibility instead of turning to the new health pattern of this generation, as the easy way out, by dieting—often result in gaining more weight than before. To reiterate, what you really need to do is to take responsibility and begin to: *Eat a well-balanced diet, exercise regularly, meditate, drink lots of water and get plenty of sleep; get regular medical check-ups—at least once a year, as part of our ongoing health lifestyle changes*, to see results.

Good health is not a destination, but a day-by-day journey, and we have that choice. We have a choice to live healthier, and that is what you will discover in this health-challenging game book. So while the lack of food can lead to disease and death, a lack of self-control management can produce **longer-term** punishable health consequences.

Most of us might not live to be 100 years, but we can learn to enjoy each day that we are given with good health practices. The *Healthiology* game is a lifestyle changing game to help you learn more about these practices, your own body and how you can prevent certain diseases from occurring or how to maintain whatever disease you already have so you can benefit from a better quality of life that is left in you.

The Power of Visualization

Visualizations are concentrated or focused intentions in the form of mental images. You think you are fat and you get fat or that you are sick and you get sick. You need to create a visualization about your health in a positive image, as strong visualization skills will provide you with a solid foundation for self-empowerment.

Stop now! Stop worrying about your size and begin to use your energy to envision about your health. The mind is very powerful and you need to use it to concentrate on the positive. The mind is like the universe. The universe is all energy, which is received and interpreted by us as information. Begin to let go of the 'too thin' or 'too fat' syndrome, to open up your good mental health balance.

Balance your life physically, emotionally and spiritually. When you do this, it will definitely allow you to improve your health by you making lifestyle changes. With lifestyle changes you will be able to see better results. Then you can begin to feel grateful for your life, as it is precious, and the only one you will ever have.

The Health Challenging Game

Not all of us will live a long time, but we can learn to live in good health each and every day. The *Healthiology 101* game is synonymous with our quality of health.

Good health is not a destination, but a day-by-day journey. It is time we take the children's health at heart, as well as our own. So this game aims to create attitudes and understanding toward nutrition, exercise, diets, digestive systems, health and diseases that will lead to healthier living. As we begin to play the game, it will help us to take responsibility for our bodies and our children's bodies, so as to help these children to take ownership from early on in life, which is healthful.

The challenge is, we know that it is hard for children to change bad eating habits, even far more than us adults do, and so what better way to get them on a good start than with a game. Both forms of the game, the book and board game is educational and fun to bring us into the reality of healthy living. So this is a tool for parents to learn and teach their children about the benefits of good health.

We are what we eat, so why not create a game that places emphasis on good health? This can be equally beneficial and enjoyed by everyone which focuses on methods of assessing what to eat, how to recognize signs of illness or symptoms of certain diseases, what to do in medical and household emergencies, how to prevent obesity and encourages exercise from a young age.

Why This Game Now

For decades, too many of us are obsessed with either '*too thin*' or '*too fat*' syndrome. This obsession is alarming and is evident in children as young as age five. The real problem we have is something much more profound—poor nutrition. Poor nutrition leads to poor health and obesity among children, teenagers, adults and the elderly. It affects all of us. Why this game now? Better late than never. The obesity numbers are increasing significantly every year, setting the tone for a generation of unfitness and chronic illnesses. Poor health and obesity often have consequences on the society resulting in health care expenditures that run into billions of dollars and are moving upward into the trillion-dollar mark. As well, no magazine would dare show us what anorexia and poor health is doing to skinny models. For poor health, it has an impact on learning disabilities, sickness, loss of productive hours, low morale and family breakdowns.

The *Healthiology 101* game is like a tour of duty. For example, clinical studies have gone as far as showing that there may be a relationship between dental problems and conditions like heart disease or even premature births. *Healthiology* watches over us and shows a commitment to helping adults and children recognized the cause of poor health and obesity. It also promotes healthy nutrition and exercise programs for economic growth and prosperity throughout its game. This health challenge game is a snapshot of what the player(s) may detect if their body is in good or poor health and what poor health can do to our bodies. We want to reverse that with good future health. *Healthiology* is trying to bring our good eating habits in line with excellent nutrition and exercise. By playing this game, we get to see firsthand what good health is all about, as well as what bad health can do to us, as demonstrated in the pages of this book.

Prevention is Better Than Having To Cure

The *Healthiology* game recognizes that there are many diseases that are avoidable, and prevention is the cornerstone. Eating the right foods and exercising prevent some diseases, and that is what this game is about to help bring awareness. Diseases will rape the body of its sight, hearing, mobility, and the use of many functions and can also cause people to experience low morale. Through this game, we give meaning to the term *prevention*, which is better than cure. By learning to play this game we are taking our health into our own precious hands; to gain the knowledge we need to foster good health.

Important Notice:

This game is no substitute for a medical doctor or therapist. This book is **not** a substitute for advice from licensed doctors or therapists. It is a book to awaken your knowledge that good health is not mere absence of disease. Regardless of medical advances and doctors, they cannot replace the individual's responsibility for every day good health practices.

This game is educational and is meant to equip us with knowledge that we can use to recognize symptoms of illnesses. The *Healthiology* game is useful for homes, workplaces, hospital recovery rooms, school groups and assignments. We can pack the book that is of dual use—reading or playing a game, on a plane ride, train, and bus, car or at home. It is a reminder that every day you need to *work* at your health in order to maintain *success*.

In practicing good health, however, one cannot emphasize the importance of: Eating a well-balanced diet (nutritiously sounding), drink lots of water for natural purification, get plenty of sleep, get at least an annual medical check up, and exercise regularly.

For exercise, find activities you like to do and do them, because that is what you will find the joy in doing. You will also find it easier to integrate the types of exercises you love into your own life. However, do <u>not</u> attempt any exercise without first consulting with your doctor.

Epidemic of the Youth

Obesity is an epidemic in America, and it is spreading like wild fire amongst children in Canada and around the world. Children are getting fat because of what food advertising they get to see on television. As been reported, in America, almost 70 percent of TV food advertising is for candies, snacks and fast food. Less and less advertising is of fruits, vegetables or diary products, making nutritional value food less attractive than junk food to children and even adults alike.

The *Healthiology* book or board game is not a humbug to brainwash you about your health. It is the 'truth' to good nutrition and exercise principles, since government and other media outlets fail to aggressively help.

According to Bill Sanders of the *New York Post*, March 29, 2007, "Youngsters between the ages of 2 and 7 see 12 food ads a day, or 4,400 ads a year; children from 8 to 12 see 21 ads a day, or 7,600 a year; teens between 13 and 17 see 17 ads a day, or 6,000 a year."

Having those concrete numbers, given by Sanders, *Healthiology* looked at youngsters to teens over a-15-year period, from ages 2 to 17, and calculated that youngsters would have watched at least 88,400 television ads, with about 2 percent, or 1,768 is nutritiously sounding and 98 percent, or 86,632 is quality-unacceptable ads. Such TV advertising ads is influential to children's obesity—as they incline to rely upon what stories those seemingly 'delicious' junk food ads imbedded in their thoughts.

Children are our greatest assets to a future life in this universe, and it is time adults help save our children from further unhealthy patterns. Do not waste another minute doing *nothing* about this problem. So how can parents help their children escape junk-ridden ads? Parents need to know that the best medicine of protecting their children's health start with them. But how can parents help their children if they do not know any better themselves? *Healthiology 101* is a health quiz game book and board game that give them the tools to do so. Parents can help children escape junk-ridden ads by doing something as simple as introducing taste buds practices.

Good Start

A good practice is never start giving a two or three-year-old child an adult food. What I mean by that is for you to never start feeding a young child with fries, donuts, cookies, candies or to give them sodas to get their taste buds acclimatized. By giving a child these foods that contain preservatives so early on in life, you are desensitizing the child's taste buds to accept these bad foods, and most of all preservative foods have salt and processed sugar in them, which are not healthy inside of the body.

For children to have an appetite for a food they have to come in contact with such food at least a dozen times. Become responsible parents and adults, and stop the epidemic and have a good start. Start your child off eating natural foods such as broccoli, tomatoes, pears or beans. You cannot go wrong eating or giving your child fruits, vegetables and whole grains, because the gift of eating from creation is the joy of making the food work for you and not you working for the food. The whole truth is if you feed your children on quality-food, junk-food ads would not interest them. Why? Because they learned from early on in life what food is good for them—eating healthy foods and also what food is bad for them—eating unhealthy foods.

Remember, we are water-based creatures, so introduce lots of water into the mix. Our bodies need water to operate most favorably—a natural purification process to maximize health. Otherwise, without plenty of water, toxin is unavoidable in the body, and that is certain to lead to overall poor health.

SECTION I

ABOUT THE STANDALONE HEALTH QUIZ

In the book the game is divided into two compartments. The first compartment is a standalone health quiz game book, where one or more players can play the game without using the board game healthy path or unhealthy ramp or moderator/scorer during playing time.

The *Healthiology* standalone health quiz game book is perfect when flying by plane or when driving on a bus, car or train, as the player(s) can self-test, record the correct or incorrect answer(s) on the health account score card and then tabulate the score at the end of playing the game.

Healthiology Guide Introduction

Healthiology 101 Guide, HG in short, is an exciting and knowledge-based, challenging healthy game. What is so good about this game is that everyone can play. It has a sequence of questions for beginners, intermediate and advanced levels. Different levels encourage us (players) not to get intimidated by the harder questions, especially when playing alone or for the first time.

Who Should Play the Quiz Game?

Anyone can play this game, but it is recommended for children as young as 8 years up to adults. Without a moderator/scorer, one player can play this game. With a moderator/scorer, two players are needed or a whole group can participate. The game has three levels, including: *Beginners, Intermediate* and *Advanced* levels so that everyone can play at their level without feeling anxious or intimidated. With the *Healthiology* game, children and parents; teacher and students or friends and co-workers, will have hours of fun playing and interacting in this stimulating game while further developing their health skills.

How to Play Health Quiz Game

Have as many as you like, alone or with others. Play the game anywhere—in bed, on a plane, train, bus, sitting at the dinner table, in a classroom or even on a beach—wherever we choose to play. If you choose to play the game with others, begin by each pulling out a number to start off the first round. One person asks the question and keep the scores if chosen to use multiple players. If, however, you are the only player, first write your answers on the score sheet and at the end of playing the game, check your answers against the answers in the back of the book to see how well you did.

The Health Quiz Game Begins

To begin the game, you must read each question and choose the correct answer of **A**, **B** or **C** from the multiple-choice questions. If you are taking the quiz game alone, you do not need a moderator/scorer.

Single Player

When playing alone, you do not need an answer card. You can play along and check your answers against the *ANSWER CHARTS* in the back of the book.

More Than One Player

Delivering the questions, the moderator/scorer will read the question to the player(s). When the moderator/scorer completes the question, giving three possible answers to the players, you have approximately 30 seconds to think about the question and come up with the correct answer.

Revealing The Correct Answers

After the 30-second, the moderator/scorer will review each answer and tell you the correct answer, while keeping a score of the players answers, and rewarding each correct answers with one hundred (100) points on the health credit section of the score card.

If, however, you answer the question incorrectly, you will receive negative one hundred (-100) points in the health debit section of the score card.

Incorrect Answers

Whenever you answer the question incorrectly, the moderator/scorer will ask you to stage a therapeutic remedial presentation in the form of exercising, singing, dancing, rapping, or reciting a poem, in fifteen seconds or less, about the danger of getting the incorrect answers. It is similar to having a headache and you need to take a pill to feel better. For example, if your answer should be C: *Eat foods low in saturated fat*, instead of A: *Eat foods high in saturated fat*, you must sing or dance to a tune with the correct answer by repeating the correct answer aloud. This is the *medication* you are going to need to get well or to get to healthier habits. This is also used to allow you to recuperate from the illness suffered, by answering the question incorrectly, in order for you to get well to continue playing in the round or consecutive rounds.

The strategy in this game is to keep on the winning circle, which is reflecting good health, not plagued by illnesses. At the end of the game, the moderator/scorer will tabulate the results and the player who was able to answer most of the questions correctly is declared the winner.

The Health Quiz Winner

The winner is acknowledged for staying healthy. Winning the *Healthiology* game requires medicinal knowledge and is an important part of self-management protocol. This game is a lifestyle game that could change your health forever!

The Health Quiz Loser

There is always a winner and a loser in a game, but there really is no loser in *Healthiology*, because playing this game will help you to learn more about the proper intake of foods, nutrition, body parts and diseases. It will help you to strive to improve healthy eating habits at home, school or otherwise, and to learn about the benefits of exercise and disease prevention. The game is a learning tool with healthy fun.

SECTION II

ABOUT THE COMPANION BOARD GAME

The second compartment is the board game. The board game is recommended for playing in groups of at least two or more players with a moderator/scorer present that will read the questions, record the answers and keep the score of each player in the game. Playing the board game, the players will also get to utilize the board by moving up or down the healthy lifestyle path or unhealthy lifestyle ramp, which is to encourage better health care nurturing.

The qualifying age to play the board game is age eight (8) to adults.

Not Just Another Board Game

Healthiology is not just another companion board game. It is a board game for teaching children and adults about lifestyle changes, i.e. health and unhealthy lifestyles. A picture tells a thousand words is what the board will remind player(s) about their health, whether they are taking good care of their health or not. They get to see how good health care or bad health can impact a person's life. As shown on the healthy lifestyle path, in nurtured health care the images are positive and showed how to prevent certain diseases and illnesses or how to look and stay younger even in golden years. On the flip side, in neglected health care the images are depressing and showed how accumulative diseases can ravage the body to even dying early before reaching the golden years.

Abstract

Healthiology, a board game for children and adults, which allow the players to see and compare good and bad health in the human body. A responsible adult can use the *Healthiology* board game to teach young children about the importance of choosing good health over bad health practices. Middle-age children can play amongst themselves, likewise, adults against adults. Alternatively, the board shows two sides, i.c. a snapshot of poor and wholesome health practices. The players get to see how poor health practices will cause many illnesses that can eventually lead to early death, while wholesome health practices will fight off many diseases and help people to live healthier and longer.

The strategy in this game is to keep on the winning path, which is on the healthy lifestyle path, by answering the questions correctly, because people practice what they are taught and learn from it.

At the end of the game, the moderator/scorer will tabulate the results and the player who was able to answer most of the questions correctly is declared the winner.

How to Play the Board Game

To begin the game (first round), the players are given three answer cards of A, B and C that they will use to display their answers. They begin the game by throwing a dice and the player with the lowest number will be player number one, and becomes the player who will lead off the game. For example, if there are four players, each player gets a 6, 4, 3 and 1 after throwing the dice; the player who throws #1 will start off the game. The name of the player will be associated with the number being displayed on the dice, example, Sam throws #1 and he becomes the first player in the game. The question will come from Beginners section and Sam gets to choose a question from any unused questions 1 through 200. The player who throws #3 will become the second player and gets to choose any unused questions from 201 through 400. The question will come from the Intermediate section. The players who throw 4 and 6 will come from the Advanced section. The player who throws dice # 4 becomes the third player and dice #6 becomes the fourth player and they both get to choose any unused questions from 401 through 800.

The moderator/score will read the question to the players, and in each round, the players are given three possible answers. (See sample question below.) For example, Sample Question:

Better eating habits are those found in children who eat:
a.   Foods low in saturated fat and high in cholesterol
b.   Foods low in saturated fat and low in cholesterol
c.   Foods high in saturated fat and low in cholesterol

How to Move on Both Sides of the Board

After throwing the dice, all the players must place the dice down at the starting point, displaying their numbers, 6, 4, 3 and 1, as that is how they will move on both sides of the board, the healthy lifestyle path or unhealthy lifestyle ramp after they have answered each of their questions correctly or incorrectly. For example, the player(s) who answered correctly (B) in the sample test question would move out of the starting point and up the healthy lifestyle path, while the player(s) who answered incorrectly would move down the unhealthy life-style ramp.

The Second and Subsequent Rounds

The player who throws # 3 will start off the second game (game 2); the third is the player who throws #4 (game 3) and the fourth player who throws #6 (game 4) will be the last player to start off the round. The players will move in this order until a player comes to the finish line of the healthy lifestyle path or the unhealthy lifestyle ramp. If there are more than one winner, the moderator/scorer must give a tie-breaking question to determine a winner or a loser.

Delivering the Questions

The moderator/scorer will read the question to the player(s). When the moderator/scorer completes the question, giving three possible answers to the players, they have approximately 30 seconds to think about the question and come up with the correct answer in their minds.

After the 30 second period is up, the moderator/scorer asks all the player(s) to pluck and drop, i.e. to pick out and place the correct answer card(s) face down on a surface, not visible to anyone else. Once the answer card is put down, the player cannot change his or her mind. They have to wait for instructions from the moderator/scorer to tell them that they must now display their cards in full view.

Revealing the Correct Answers

The correct sample question answer is B. The player(s) who gets the correct answer will earn one hundred (+100) points on the healthy lifestyle path and get to record the score under the health credit section on the score card. However, if the player(s) gets an incorrect answer, he or she would earn negative one hundred (-100) points backward down on the healthy lifestyle path and get to record the score under the health debit section on the score card. A round up on the unhealthy lifestyle ramp, the player(s) would move negative one hundred points forward on the unhealthy lifestyle ramp. When landing on the healthy path, the player(s) would move positive one hundred points forward on the healthy lifestyle path.

Landing on the Healthy Lifestyle Path

Whenever a player lands on the healthy lifestyle path, they get 'positive' 100 points and move forward. The player to reach the finish line is paid a check for $1,000 and the game will start all over, from the beginning, with all the players throwing out the dice to begin a fresh round of play.

Landing on the healthy lifestyle path and to move from the healthy lifestyle path to the unhealthy lifestyle ramp, the player(s) would move negative one hundred (-100) points backward. However, if on the unhealthy lifestyle ramp the player(s) would still receive 'negative' 100 points, but continue to move forward on the unhealthy lifestyle ramp. To move backward when on the unhealthy lifestyle ramp, the player(s) must answer a question correctly.

Landing on the Unhealthy Lifestyle Ramp

Whenever a player lands on the unhealthy lifestyle ramp, the player will get 'negative' 100 points. The moderator/scorer will ask the player(s) to stage a therapeutic remedial presentation in the form of exercising, singing, dancing, rapping, or recite a poem, in fifteen seconds or less, about the danger of the disease landed on. This is the *medication* the player(s) requires to recuperate from the illness suffered, in order to continue playing in the round or consecutive rounds.

During the game, if a player who has been on the healthy lifestyle path comes up with an incorrect answer, he or she would take a step backward. If the player(s) continues to lose and comes to the end of the healthy lifestyle path, then he or she must move down to the unhealthy lifestyle ramp, which is equated to losing one hundred points, per incorrect answered question. When a player(s) who has been on the unhealthy lifestyle ramp comes up with the correct answer, he or she would take steps backward, which is also a positive forward step, to add one hundred points towards the health credit account. If, however, the player on the unhealthy lifestyle ramp continues to lose in ten consecutive games, he or she would come to the end of the unhealthy lifestyle ramp, which is a cemetery. At this point, the player(s) is pronounced dead, and, therefore, is automatically out of the game and must hand over any cash already won, and has to wait for the first player to reach the winner's line (healthy lifestyle path) to begin a brand new round or all other players to end their rounds, in the cemetery's line (unhealthy lifestyle ramp), to begin a brand new round of the game.

Automatic Expulsion from the Game

When a player(s) has reached the unhealthy ramp cemetery, the player(s) is pronounced dead and is automatically expelled from the game. The player(s) must hand over any cash already won, and at this point must wait for a player to come to the winner's line of the healthy lifestyle path to get back into the game or all the players in the game have ended at the cemetery's line of the unhealthy lifestyle ramp.

Automatic expulsion is given to every player that reaches the cemetery's line of the unhealthy lifestyle ramp. If all the players reach the cemetery's line a new round of game must begin. However on the healthy lifestyle path, the first player to reach the winner's line will automatically start a new round of that game. Remember, a new game cannot be enforced until the first player reaches the winner's line, or all the players reach the cemetery's line, to begin a fresh new round.

To End the Board Game

At the end of playing the game, all the player's points are tabulated to decide a winner and a loser. The player with the highest score will be declared the winner and would get to keep all the money he or she already won plus a bonus check. The loser(s) will look in the eyes of the moderator/scorer and say, "I'm not as healthy as I thought."

The Board Game Winner

The first player to get to the finish line with the highest score would receive, in addition to the money already won during the playing of the game, a bonus check for $50,000, to sail away on their own private boat, into the sunset. If there is more than one winner to reach the finish line, there will be a tie-breaking question, as there can only be one winner in this game.

Winning the *Healthiology* health challenge check requires medicinal knowledge and is an important part of self-management protocol. This game is a lifestyle game that could change your health forever!

The Board Game Loser

There is always a winner and a loser in a game, and in the *Healthiology* game, the loser(s) with the lowest score to end the round is pronounced dead, and therefore leaves with nothing. There really is no loser, however, because playing this game will help the players to learn more about the proper intake of foods, nutrition, their body parts, symptoms, diseases and the lack of exercise consequences.

About Winning or Losing

We hope that winning or losing will help the players strive to improve healthy eating habits at home, school or otherwise, and to learn about exercise benefits and disease prevention. The *Healthiology* game is a learning tool with much healthy fun in it.

SECTION III

The Beginners questions are 1 through 200. Good luck!

BEGINNERS QUESTIONS

1.   Another name for abdominal pain is:
   a. Head/brain pain
   b. Stomach/belly pain
   c. Jaw/gum pain

2.   A child who is immune to something means that the child is:
   a. Free to expose
   b. Free to catch
   c. protected from

3.   The answer that best describes when an accident can happen:
   a. At anytime
   b. Rush hour
   c. When you are not paying attention

4.   Acne is a:
   a. Bowel disorder
   b. Skin disorder
   c. Neck disorder

5.   The best predictor of how long you will live is to:
   a. Walk 30 minutes a day
   b. Sleep 5 hours a night
   c. Eat foods that contain saturated and trans fat

6.   Fractures are:
   a. Swollen bones
   b. Broken bones
   c. Swollen cicatrix

7.   Asthma is a:
       a. Toy for babies
       b. Lung disease
       c. Stomach pain

8.   Foods with the following ingredients should be avoided:
       a. Enriched flour, fructose corn syrup, saturated and trans fat
       b. Whole wheat flour, protein, fiber and 100% whole grains
       c. None of the above

9.   The most common allergic disorder is:
       a. Hay fever
       b. Food
       c. Bronchial asthma

10.   Arthritis is caused by:
       a. Pain in a joint
       b. Inflammation of a joint
       c. Infection in the knee joint

11.   Rheumatoid arthritis is more common in:
       a. Hot climates
       b. Rainy climates
       c. Cool climates

12.   Everyone who has symptoms of a heart attack should:
       a. Lay flat on your back and go to sleep
       b. Call 911
       c. Drive yourself to the emergency room

13.   Asthma sufferers usually experience:
       a. Irregular coughs
       b. Wheezing and short of breath
       c. Wheezing

14.   The healthiest foods to eat from these groups are:
       a. Spinach, fries and sodas
       b. Fried chicken, white bread and juice
       c. Steamed broccoli, beans and milk

15.   Bronchitis usually occurs following a:
      a. Common rash
      b. Common cold
      c. Common heartburn

16.   Choose the drink with the best ingredients:
      a. Filtered water, high fructose corn syrup, orange juice concentrate
      b. Carbonated water, high fructose corn syrup, citric acid, natural flavors
      c. 100% pure orange juice, filtered water, concentrated cherry juice

17.   Stroke happens at all ages, but is:
      a. Greater risk in young children
      b. Greater risk in older people
      c. No risk at all

18.   People who are overweight generally have a:
      a. High metabolism
      b. Low metabolism
      c. Density of growth

19.   Bedsore is an ulcer of the skin resulting from:
      a. The condition of the mattress
      b. Lying on hard bed surfaces
      c. Prolonged stay in bed

20.   A benign tumor is:
      a. Harmless, not malignant
      b. Outlook of the tumor is favorable
      c. All of the above (A & B)

21.   You need to get an average of:
      a. 25 grams of fiber every day
      b. 72 grams of fiber every day
      c. 90 grams of fiber every day

22.   Biceps referred to:
      a. Weak muscle in the knuckle
      b. Strong muscle of the upper arm
      c. Strong muscle of the lower arm

23.   Another name for Acne is:
       a. Serum
       b. Face deformity
       c. Blackhead

24.   Blindness can be:
       a. Partial, fractional or obese
       b. Total or partial, temporary or permanent
       c. Partial or permanent, natural or supernatural

25.   Blood clotting is the defense against:
       a. Blood spots
       b. Blood veins
       c. Bleeding

26.   Hypertension is often called "the silent killer" because it normally has:
       a. No symptoms
       b. Numerous symptoms
       c. Minor symptoms

27.   Types of asthmas are:
       a. Allergy asthma and bronchitis asthma
       b. Allergy asthma and detective asthma
       c. Allergy asthma and non-allergic asthma

28.   The correct name for High Blood Pressure is:
       a. Hyperextension
       b. Hypertension
       c. Systolic blood pressure

29.   A blood test is done to:
       a. Detect if someone has high blood pressure
       b. Detect if fatty deposits are around the heart
       c. Detect many different diseases

30.   Tips to fight the common cold and flu are:
       a. Cover mouth and nose when coughing or sneezing, wash hands, drink fluids, eat fruits and vegetables
       b. Uncover mouth and nose to spray out sneeze, eat fruits and exercise
       c. Lay in bed for at least three days during the incubation period and drink fluids

31.   The bowel holds the:
       a. Digestive system
       b. Femur
       c. Asphyxia system

32.   The human brain is protected by:
       a. Hair and scalp
       b. Thick bones of the skull
       c. Thin bones of the skull

33.   The brain is a mass of:
       a. Nerve cells and nerve fibers
       b. Nerve cells and skull
       c. Never fibers and skull

34.   Salt makes you:
       a. Lose weight
       b. Gain weight
       c. Sweat a lot

35.   Brain damage can be caused by:
       a. Birth injuries and concussion
       b. Circulatory changes in the brain
       c. All of the above (A & B)

36.   Bronchitis is a:
       a. High fever
       b. A form of muscle pain
       c. Coughing sickness

37.   Bronchopneumonia is a form of:
       a. Pneumonia
       b. Brucellosis
       c. Hay fever

38.   What is the correct answer as stated for medical casualty in the United States:
       a. One in every three women will die from heart attack
       b. One in every five women will die from heart attack
       c. One in every ten women will die from heart attack

39.   The different types of burns are:
       a. Minor-degree burns and first-degree burns
       b. First, second and third degrees burns
       c. First, second, third, forth and fifth degrees burns

40.   First-degree burns show:
       a. Dark color on the surface of the skin
       b. Tissue exposure of the skin
       c. Redness of the unbroken skin

41.   A dermatologist is a:
       a. Skin specialist
       b. Bone specialist
       c. Lungs specialist

42.   Caffeine does the following:
       a. It is given to patients suffering from Angina
       b. It stimulates the muscles of a person who suffers from a stroke
       c. It stimulates the heart, nervous system and kidney

43.   Calcium is not only good for bones and teeth but is essential to:
       a. Blood clotting
       b. Blood transfusion
       c. Migraine pain

44.   Nutritional supplements should not be used as a substitute for:
       a. Fighting a common cold
       b. Healthy diet
       c. None of the above

45. An eating disorder that is not easily detected is:
    c. Couch eating
    b. Hallow eating
    c. Binge eating

46. The acronym PET in science stands for:
    a. Physical Exercise Treatment
    b. Positron Emission Topography
    c. Physical Energy Topology

47. The procedure that allows doctors to observe chemical and metabolism process in motion is called a:
    a. PET scan
    b. Eclampsia scan
    c. Positron scan

48. Callus is a common:
    a. Gum disorder
    b. Stomach disorder
    c. Foot disorder

49. The adult liver is:
    a. The body's smallest organ
    b. The body's largest organ
    c. The body's smallest vessel

50. Delay in seeking treatment of cancer causes it to:
    a. become dormant
    b. become fatal
    c. spread to the skin

51. Laughter is often referred to as:
    a. Life's lubricant
    b. Life's happiness
    c. Life's sadness

52.   Cancer is:
    a. Neither contagious, transmittable nor communicable
    b. Neither infectious, catching nor transferable
    c. All of the above (A & B)

53.   When someone gets 'car sickness' it means the person is experiencing:
    a. Dizziness, vomiting and nausea
    b. Vomiting and tiredness
    c. None of the above

54.   'Car sickness' is most common among:
    a. Animals
    b. Young children
    c. Old people

55.   Malignant tumors are:
    a. Benign
    b. Cancerous
    c. Small Bunions

56.   Cells are found in:
    a. Living things and plants
    b. Human and animal
    c. All of the above (A & B)

57.   Chemotherapy treatment is given to:
    a. Cancer patients
    b. Chicken pox patients
    c. Heart patients

58.   Chicken pox symptoms are:
    a. Slight fever, mild discomfort and skin irritation
    b. Little raised pimples on the skin, faced body and scalp
    c. All of the above (A & B)

59.   Diabetes can be:
    a. Prevented
    b. Delayed
    c. All of the above (A & B)

60.   Coffee contains caffeine, which is a:
       a. Colitis
       b. Stimulant
       c. Vitamin E

61.   Cold sore is a:
       a. Fluid that presents itself around the mouth
       b. Rash on the skin
       c. Mild virus infection that appears on the mouth

62.   Colic is a:
       a. Depositary of belching
       b. Severe, cramping, gripping, pain
       c. Associated with dizziness

63.   Color blindness is the:
       a. Ability to tell the differences between colors
       b. Inability to recognize lighter colors
       c. Inability to differentiate between colors

64.   Dandruff consists of:
       a. Large scabs formed on the hair
       b. Little scales of skin formed on the scalp
       c. Noticeable scales usually found in the center of the head

65.   Dandruff is marked by:
       a. Itching in the head, falling out of hair and lusterless hair
       b. Falling out of hair and thinning of hair
       c. Healthy looking hair

66.   Ordinary dandruff can be removed from the scalp by:
       a. Washing or shampooing the hair slightly
       b. Washing or shampooing hair thoroughly
       c. Trimming the hair down to a low cut

67.   When prostate cancer is detected in time, the cure rate of the person is:
       a. Low
       b. Moderate
       c. High

68.   To help manage pain you can enhance your body's immune system by:
        a. Humor
        b. Drinking a cup of coffee every day
        c. Complaining about the pain and taking pills

69.   In the United States of America, approximately:
        a. approximately 50,000 women are diagnosed with breast cancer each year
        b. approximately 200,000 women are diagnosed with breast cancer each year
        c. approximately 500,000 women are diagnosed with breast cancer each year

70.   Dizziness is the:
        a. Sensation that makes you feel like you are whirling around
        b. Sensation that one is ready to fall asleep
        c. Sensation that one is dozing off

71.   A toddler can:
        a. Use a glass
        b. Use knife and fort
        c. Use a spoon and cup

72.   Disinfectants are agents that:
        a. Revive disease-producing microbes inside the body
        b. Kill disease-producing microbes outside the body
        c. Entertain disease-producing microbes outside the body

73.   The best way to take care of your inner ear is to:
        a. Use a q-tip to clean them
        b. Syringe them
        c. Leave them alone

74.   Earache may be due to:
        a. Wax and foreign bodies inside the ear
        b. Inflammation
        c. All of the above (A & B)

75. EENT stands for:
    a. Eyes, eardrums, nostrils and thorax
    b. Eye, ear, nose and throat
    c. Effusion, ego, nausea and thumb

76. Doing regular exercise cuts the heart disease by about:
    a. 2 percent
    b. 10 percent
    c. 25 percent

77. To be in a trance means that you are:
    a. Dozing off
    b. Half-asleep, half-awake
    c. Sleep walking

78. When you exercise the best way to know if it is effective is:
    a. How you look
    b. How you feel
    c. How many pounds you lost

79. The most important meal of the day is:
    a. Breakfast
    b. Lunch
    c. Dinner

80. The eyes are protected by being in the sockets within the bones of the skull and by the:
    a. Eyelids and iris
    b. Eyelids and pupil
    c. Eyelids and eyelashes

81. The eye has:
    a. No muscles inside
    b. No sclera or muscles inside
    c. Muscle inside

82.   A black eye is:
        a. Known as cross-eye
        b. a bruise in the eye area
        c. An infection in the eye

83.   Fainting is a:
        a. Undeviating loss of consciousness
        b. Temporary loss of consciousness
        c. Permanent loss of consciousness

84.   Common foot troubles are:
        a. Pressure points, high heels, low arches
        b. Calluses, corns, bunions, blisters
        c. Low arches, calluses, pressure points

85.   Fumigation is the process of:
        a. Accumulation of insects
        b. Destroying insects
        c. Harvesting of animals

86.   Fungicide is anything that:
        a. Kills weeds
        b. Kills airborne
        c. Kills fungi or fungus

87.   Growing pains is:
        a. A myth
        b. Pain in children
        c. A cliché referring to baby animals

88.   Human hair usually grows about:
        a. An inch in 6 weeks
        b. An inch in 12 weeks
        c. An inch in 24 weeks

89.   Whooping cough is:
        a. A minor cough
        b. A minor adult disease
        c. A serious childhood disease

90.   The acronym WMA stands for:
       a. Workers Medical Adjustment
       b. World Medical Association
       c. World Medical Assessment

91   Headache is a:
       a. Disease
       b. Infection
       c. Symptom

92.   A family doctor is a physician who engages in:
       a. Skin diseases
       b. Delivery of newborn babies in the children's ward
       c. General practice of medicine

93.   A running ear is a sign of:
       a. Hard wax lodged in the eardrum
       b. Chronic infection
       c. Foreign bodies lodged in the eardrum

94.   MRI is the acronym for:
       a. Management Resource Information
       b. Medicare Resource Index
       c. Magnetic Resonance Imaging

95.   Dizziness is a:
       a. Disease of the inner ear
       b. Disease of the brain
       c. Mild feelings of the ear

96.   MRI is:
       a. Painful
       b. Painless
       c. Chronic

97.   Heartburn is a:
       a. Heart pain experienced from poorly chewed food
       b. Heartbeats with rapid pulsation
       c. Burning sensation in the food tube (esophagus)

98.   Heartburn has to do with:
         a. burning in the heart
         b. indigestion marked by a burning sensation in the esophagus
         c. the nicotine from smoking

99.   Heroin is a:
         a. Male sex organ
         b. Narcotic drug
         c. Irritation of the skull

100.   Influenza is also known as:
         a. Flu or grippe
         b. Flu or fusion
         c. Influenza or radio waves

101.   The jaw bone is the:
         a. Bones that connect to the tongue
         b. Bones that connects the jaw to the head
         c. Bones that hold the teeth

102.   Where the bones of the body fit together, these are known as:
         a. Joints
         b. Muscles
         c. Ligaments

103.   Intoxication means either:
         a. Drunkenness or hallucination
         b. Drunkenness or unconsciousness
         c. Drunkenness or poisoning

104.   Insects are:
         a. Both friends and enemies of man
         b. Both foe and enemies of man
         c. Both friends and ally of man

105.   Lice infest the:
         a. Hair only
         b. Body, hair and clothing
         c. Arm pit, body and bedding

106.   Malaria is a:
a. Bedbug-borne disease
b. Mosquito-borne disease
c. Lice-borne disease

107.   Menstruation occurs normally in a:
a. Boy's late teens
b. Girl's late teens
c. Girl's early teens

108   The best defense against illness is:
a. Your immune system working at optimum level
b. Your motion in place
c. Eat lots of fruits and drink plenty of water

109.   The acronym MS stands for:
a. Major surgery
b. Minor surgery
c. Multiple Sclerosis

110.   Abnormal reddish coloration or blotch on some parts of the skin is a:
a. Freckle
b. Acne
c. Rash

111.   A popular term for injection is:
a. Scarlet
b. Shots
c. Tetanus

112.   FDA is the acronym for:
a. Federal and Democratic Administration
b. Food and Drug Administration
c. Food and Drug Association

113.   CDC is the acronym for:
a. Children Dietary Center
b. Calorie Deficiency Cells
c. Center for Disease Control

114.   Vegetables that contain chlorophyll, which detoxifies and rejuvenates
        the liver, kidney and colon are:
        a. Cabbage, lettuce, broccoli and watercress
        b. Carrot, mushroom, Eggplant and watercress
        c. Broccoli, grape, carrot and calcium

115.   The human body has:
        a. 108 bones
        b. 160 bones
        c. 206 bones

116.   The process of digestion begins with:
        a. Mouth
        b. Stomach
        c. Intestine

117.   A baby crawls at what age?
        a. About three months
        b. About six months
        c. About nine months

118.   A diaper change should be:
        a. Once a day
        b. After every feeding
        c. Whenever the baby is wet

119.   Down syndrome occurs at:
        a. Fertilization
        b. Birth
        c. After birth up to age one

120.   BMD is the acronym for:
        a. Bone Management Department
        b. Bone Mineral Density
        c. Biopsy Miracle Drug

121.   SIDS is also known as:
   a. Capillaries
   b. Crib death
   c. Twilight sleep

122.   Your child's nutrition is important for:
   a. Growing between one and twelve
   b. Overall health
   c. Gaining weight

123.   The acronym WHO stands for:
   a. World Health Organization
   b. Workers Hippocratic Oath
   c. Witch Hazel Ointment

124.   To have an abscess is to:
   a. Have a fever
   b. Have a painful toothache
   c. Have an accumulation of pus

125.   If someone gets an abrasion you will see:
   a. Rubbing or scraping off of skin
   b. A large cut under the feet
   c. a toe nail is missing

126.   The abdomen has the following organs:
   a. Stomach, femur and heart
   b. Spinal cord, liver and stomach
   c. Stomach, liver and spleen

127.   To stop the bleeding on someone's hand is to:
   a. Place hand in cold water and let it remain there for two minutes
   b. Wrap hand with clean warm towel and let it relax
   c. Wrap hand with clean towel and apply pressure

128.   When an acidic stomach has too much residue, it creates the symptoms of:
   a. Heartburn
   b. Pain and upset stomach
   c. Heartburn, belching and pain

129.   To have an acute abdominal pain is:
        a. Severe pain a.
        b. A mild pain
        c. A moderate pain

130.   The abbreviation of water is:
        a. H1o
        b. H2o
        c. H3o

131.   On an average, menstruation occurs every:
        a. 16 days
        b. 28 days
        c. 38 days

132.   The meaning of MD is:
        a. Doctor of Divinity
        b. Manageable Dosage
        c. Doctor of Medicine

133.   Ball and socket joints are found in the:
        a. Shoulders
        b. Stomach
        c. Legs

134.   Another name for immunization is:
        a. Illusion
        b. Vaccination
        c. Hallucination

135.   A normal menstrual period may lasts for:
        a. 3 to 5 days
        b. 5 to 7 days
        c. 7 to 9 days

136.   Mumps swelling usually begins:
        a. Under the neck and spreads spontaneously
        b. On one side and spreads to the other in two weeks
        c. On both sides and spreads and enlarge in a few days

137. An unsettled feeling of being sick at the stomach and ready to vomit is
      called:
      a. Colic
      b. Nausea
      c. Belching

138. The nose communicate with the:
      a. Eyes, ears and throat
      b. Mouth and throat
      c. Nose, ears and throat

139. A running nose is usually a sign of:
      a. An influenza or breathing problem
      b. A common flu or hay fever
      c. Breathing problems

140. In colds and hay fever stuffy nose is usually followed by:
      a. Low appetite
      b. Sleepiness
      c. running nose

141. Calculus is a:
      a. Calcium deposits to the body
      b. Branch of science research
      c. Stone formed in the body

142. Cancer is:
      a. A contagious disease
      b. A group of many diseases
      c. A single cell disease

143. A babies or teens need:
      a. Active, physical play for at least 30 minutes every day
      b. Active, mental play for at least 10 hours every day
      c. Inactive, physical play using a video game for at least 3 hours every day

144.   In the United States, childhood obesity has:
        a. Slightly gone up in the last 20 years
        b. Gone up around 2% in the last 20 years
        c. Doubled in the last 20 years

145.   Carbon monoxide (CO) is a:
        a. Highly poisonous gas
        b. Colorless and odorless gas
        c. All of the above (A & B)

146.   Cardiac refers to:
        a. The mouth
        b. The heart
        c. The cardiovascular nerve

147.   A cardiologist is someone with a profession as a:
        a. Heart specialist
        b. Lungs specialist
        c. Brain specialist

148.   MMA is the acronym for:
        a. Medicare Modernization Act
        b. Medical Malpractice Administration
        c. Medicare Management Association

149.   ADA is the acronym for:
        a. American Disabilities Association
        b. American Disabilities Administration
        c. Americans with Disabilities Act

150.   SIDS is the acronym for:
        a. Sulfonamide Infant Drugs Supplement
        b. Sudden Infant Death Syndrome
        c. Skin Inflammation Detected by Sunlight

151.   Long-term exposure to ultraviolet (UV) rays can lead to:
        a. Cataracts and macular degeneration
        b. People wearing contact lenses
        c. Does no known harm to humans

152.   GI is the acronym for:
a. Gastrointestinal
b. Goodwin Institute
c. Glutamic Indigestion

153.   Alcohol is a:
a. Tonic
b. Depressant drug
c. 'Buoy up' drug

154.   The most common allergy disorders are:
a. Hives, hay fever and skin blemish
b. Food, hives, bronchial asthma and drug rashes
c. Hay fever, eczema, food, hives and drug rashes

155.   Alopecia is associated with:
a. Baldness
b. Thin hairline
c. Patches of hair

156.   To have amnesia, means someone suffers from a:
a. Miscarriage
b. Loss of memory
c. Broken vein

157.   Medical problems are:
a. Illnesses, diseases or injuries that do not necessarily require surgery
b. Illnesses, diseases or injuries that require surgery
c. Illnesses, diseases or injuries that need a psychiatrist to assess

158.   The causes of diabetes is:
a. Low cholesterol levels
b. Too much fatty acids
c. The inability of the pancreas to produce enough insulin to break
down fat for absorption into the body

159.   A slump posture may indicate that the person is:
        a. Very happy
        b. Suffers from a bone disorder
        c. Not happy or not feeling well

160.   Tropical diseases are associated with:
        a. Black water fever, dengue, cholera and yaws
        b. Dengue, cholera, rabbit fever and typhoid fever
        c. Rabbit fever, typhoid fever, tuberculosis and trichomoniasis

161.   The destruction of skin or mucous membrane, with or without infection or pain is called:
        a. Trichiasis
        b. Gallbladder
        c. An ulcer

162.   The lined tube that carries urine from the bladder outside the body is:
        a. Urethra
        b. Uterus
        c. Vagina

163.   Another name for urination is:
        a. Bloating
        b. Micturition
        c. Urinary tract

164.   Abscess is formed from:
        a. Nitrogen and oxygen mixed
        b. Infected, broken-down tissues
        c. Saliva and nitrogen under the gum

165.   Abscesses can appear in what parts of the body:
        a. Roots of the teeth and eye
        b. Roots of the teeth, in the ear and liver
        c. In the eye and intestine

166.   When you locate an accident victim that is not breathing, you give:
a. Artificial respiration
b. The victim an aspirin
c. Place the victim on their back

167.   Another name for Acetylsalicylic acid is:
a. Aspirin
b. Miscarriage
c. Adrenalin

168.   Ascorbic acid is known as:
a. Protein
b. Vitamin C
c. Vitamin D

169.   Fatigue is a:
a. Tired feeling
b. Happy feeling
c. Sleepy feeling

170.   Acetic acid is the acid in:
a. Ammonia
b. Vinegar
c. Carbon monoxide

171.   Healthy ways to eat meat or meat substitutes include:
a. Broil, grill, steam, roast, stew or stir-fry
b. Grill, steam, stew, cook or deep-fry
c. Stew, steam, roast, barbecue, brown or fry

172.   Adrenalin is also referred to as the:
a. Rush
b. Emergency hormone
c. Hyperemia

173.   Obesity is caused by an individual eating:
a. Less food than the average person
b. More drinking and less food than is necessary
c. More food than is necessary

174. Obese children need:
    a. Less food and more activity than their peers
    b. More food and more activity than their peers
    c. Less food and less activity than their peers

175. Caries referred to:
    a. Lungs decay
    b. Blindness
    c. Bone decay

176. Another name for chicken pox is:
    a. Renal artery
    b. Vertebra
    c. Varicella

177. Chicken pox is a common:
    a. Childhood disease caused by a specific virus
    b. Childhood disease caused by mosquito bites
    c. Childhood disease caused by vein disruption

178. Each year, in America, a number of people developed the flu, approximately how many?
    a. 10 million
    b. 40 million
    c. 75 million

179. The best answer for the number of people in America with anorexia is:
    a. 2 million
    b. 8 million
    c. None of the above

180. The best foods to eat are those that contain:
    a. Trans fat, saturated fat or high cholesterol levels
    b. No saturated fat, no trans fat or low cholesterol levels
    c. Sodium, cholesterol, trans fat or saturated fat

181. Choose the best group of foods below:
      a. Broccoli, carrots, fish, brown rice and skim milk
      b. French fries, hamburger, pop and gravy
      c. Baked potatoes, sour cream, white rice and custard

182. Caffeine is a:
      a. Fluid that comes cooking with peppers
      b. Cough medicine
      c. Stimulating drug present in coffee, tea and soda pop

183. What is the best source needed for growing children:
      a. High fat, low mineral and high low source of iron
      b. Calcium, low fat and excellent source of iron
      c. Calcium only

184. Which best describes the lack of exercise and to what it may be related:
      a. Poor health
      b. Poor dressing
      c. Poor speech

185. People who do not smoke:
      a. Can get cancer
      b. Cannot get cancer
      c. None of the above

186. A major factor of heart disease is:
      a. Lack of sleep
      b. Smoking
      c. Lack of exercise

187. Proper nutrition can also prevent:
      a. Pregnancy
      b. Living longer
      c. Many medical problems

188.   Malnutrition is the:
    a. Failure to receive candies
    b. Failure to receive adequate nourishment
    c. Failure to receive 50 calories intake per day

189.   Cleanliness and skin care are needed for:
    a. Comfort, safety and health
    b. Health and spasm
    c. Comfort, image and tone

190.   The foods that provide the most protein are:
    a. Leeks, tomatoes and mustards
    b. Fries, cookies and cheese
    c. Beans, meats and fish

191.   One of the proper and best ways to protect against natural defense is to:
    a. Avoid eating too many junk food
    b. Wash hands
    c. Eat only foods containing fiber

192.   Nutrition is important for children:
    a. Between one and twelve
    b. Overall health
    c. Adding on extra weight

193.   Fruits such as grapefruits, oranges, lemons, tomatoes and limes are best source of:
    a. Olive oil
    b. Vitamin C
    c. Vitamin D

194.   The best way to get rid of obesity is to:
    a. Increase diet and get plenty of sleep
    b. Exercise for 15 minutes before eating and increase your diet
    c. Reduce food intake and exercise

195. To get kids to become mindful of movement and motor skills, they should:
    a. Run, sleep or eat fatty food
    b. Walk, run dance or throw a ball
    c. Walk, eat high fats or high cholesterol

196. Healthy eating habits and regular exercise should be:
    a. A regular part of your family's life
    b. An uncommon part of your family's life
    c. A minimal part of your school's extra curriculum activities

197. Common reactions to the Statins medicine when mixed with grape-fruit juice is:
    a. Lower blood levels of the medicine
    b. No reaction is known to doctors
    c. Higher blood levels of the medicine

198. Diabetes medicines mixed with alcohol will cause:
    a. Rapid heartbeat and blood pressure changes
    b. No rapid heartbeat or blood pressure changes occur
    c. Synchronizing heart and valve changes

199. At age 65, men and women absorb less calcium, and, therefore, would need:
    a. 600 mg calcium and 100 IU Vitamin D per day
    b. 1,200 mg calcium and 400 IU Vitamin D per day
    c. 1,000 mg calcium every other day

200. Bad fats are saturated fats and trans fats; good fats are:
    a. Monounsaturated fats and polyunsaturated fats
    b. Monosaturated fats and polysaturated fats
    c. None of the above are good fats

SECTION IV

This is the Intermediate section, questions 201 through to 400. Good luck!

INTERMEDIATE
QUESTIONS

201. A person needs at least:
   a. One bowel movement every other day
   b. Two bowel movements every day
   c. Occasionally

202. Bulimia eating disorder is caused by:
   a. Drug inhaling or self-induced vomiting
   b. Over exercise, malnutrition or dieting
   c. Binge eating, dieting, laxative or self-induced vomiting

203 The best answer to Multiple Sclerosis (MS) cure should be:
   a. MS can only be cured and managed in young adults
   b. MS can be cured by given the proper medication
   c. MS cannot be cured but it can be managed

204. Fill in the correct blanks: esophageal, liver, lung, uterine, prostate, is related to:
   a. Pancreatic caner
   b. Pancreatic emphysema
   c. Pancreatic pneumonia

205. Diabetes occurs when which organs does not work properly:
   a. Kidney
   b. Coronary
   c. Pancreas

206.   The *"sunshine vitamin"* which *is* essential to the utilization of calcium and phosphorus, especially in proper bone and tooth formation is found in:
a. Vitamin C
b. Vitamin D
c. Vitamin E

207.   The words '*Angina Pectoris*' mean:
a. Pain or strangling in the chest
b. Wheezing or strangling in the chest
c. Weakness of breaths or wheezing

208.   When someone is suffering from anorexia it means that the person has:
a. Plenty of appetite for food
b. Appetite for liquids only
c. No appetite for food

209.   Overgrowth of fungus called *Candida*, which is usually present in small amounts in the vagina, is a:
a. Venereal diseases
b. Suffocating vaginal pains
c. Yeast infections

210.   Canker signs is a:
a. Sores that does not heal, usually in the mouth, tongue or lips
b. Pains that is aching, usually around the breast and stomach
c. Swelling of the breast and stomach, usually before your sinuses

211.   Carbon monoxide when breathed into the lungs:
a. Replaces oxygen and decreases carbon monoxide poisoning
b. Restores oxygen and decreases carbon monoxide poisoning
c. Displaces oxygen and can cause carbon monoxide poisoning

212.   To care for someone with carbon monoxide poisoning, the person should:
a. Get fresh air and get medical help
b. Apply artificial respiration if breathing has stopped;
c. All of the above (A & B)

213. Some types of illness that may affect a diabetic person includes:
      a. Smoking, obesity or stress
      b. Flu, sore throat or foot infection
      c. Exercise, heart trouble or insulin

214. The healthy ways to eat starch:
      a. Eat cereal with 1% milk, whole grain breads or cereals
      b. Eat cereal with 2% milk, white bread or pastries
      c. Eat cereals with evaporated milk, tortilla chips or pretzels

215. When you are allergic to something, it means your body reacts:
      a. Negatively to something you eat, smell or is present in the environment
      b. Positively to something you eat, smell or the environment
      c. Negatively to coughing, wheezing or sneezing

216. The 4th cause of death around the world is:
      a. Cardiac arrest (heart attack)
      b. Diabetes
      c. AIDS (acquired immunodeficiency syndrome)

217. Castration of a male means:
      a. The removal of the ovaries
      b. The removal of an infection
      c. The removal of the testicles

218. Vitamin ... boosts the red blood cells, promotes maintenance and growth tissues and helps maintain nerve cells:
      a. B5
      b. B12
      c. B24

219. Catalepsy is a:
      a. Strange state of the muscular rigidity
      b. The patient does not move from whatever position he or she has been placed in
      c. All of the above (A & B)

220.   Cataract is:
   a. Clouding of the crystalline lens of the eyes
   b. The fullness of the eye lens
   c. The operation process to remove a cataract

221.   Cataract is the:
   a. Darkness around the iris of the eye
   b. Watering of the lens of the eye
   c. Clouding of the crystalline lens of the eye

222.   Cancer signs is a:
   a. Painless lump, thickening in the breast or elsewhere
   b. Any change in size or color of a mole or wart
   c. All of the above (A & B)

223.   Carbon monoxide has a:
   a. Weaker affinity than oxygen for the blood flowing to the veins
   b. Stronger affinity than oxygen for the hemoglobin of the red blood cells
   c. Weaker similarity than oxygen for the hemoglobin of the white blood cells

224.   Testicular cancer is a painless lump in the:
   a. Testicle or a heavy, swollen scrotum
   b. Testicle or a heavy, swollen cervix
   c. Testicle or a heavy, swollen breast

225.   Causes of high blood sugar (hyperglycemia):
   a. Not enough water and too much exercise
   b. Delayed meal and not enough insulin
   c. Not enough insulin and too much food

226.   Anoxia is:
   a. The lack of appetite
   b. Too little oxygen reaching the tissues
   c. Too little oxygen in the blood stream

227.   If you feel that someone is getting an attack of appendicitis what is the
        recommended action at this time:
        a. Drink a glass of cold water
        b. Take a laxative
        c. Eat nothing

228.   To be feeling acrocyanosis is to be:
        a. Cold
        b. Hot
        c. Warm

229.   An Artery is a:
        a. Blood type
        b. Blood vessel that carries the blood away from the heart
        c. Vein that carries the blood to the heart

230.   The person who is likely to get rheumatoid arthritis:
        a. Women and men
        b. Children
        c. All of the above (A & B)

231.   Rheumatoid arthritis usually starts with:
        a. Pain in the head
        b. Stomach pain and stiffness in the feet
        c. Weakness and pain in the hands

232.   Someone who dies from asphyxia is:
        a. Choked to death
        b. Drowned to death
        c. Mauled to death

233.   The major prevention of heart attacks and strokes could be prevented
        by controlling:
        a. Amount of food intake, diet and exercise
        b. Examination of the body fluids flouting over the heart
        c. Cholesterol, blood pressure and cigarette smoking

234.   Bacteria come in many different sizes, but in these principal shapes:
    a. Rod or pencil-shaped, spherical or dot-shaped
    b. Spiral or comma-shaped
    c. All of the above (A & B)

235.   Genetic diseases are transmitted from parent to child through the:
    a. Genes
    b. Fallopian tubes
    c. Breasts feeding

236.   Blackheads are associated with:
    a. Men and baldness
    b. Adolescence
    c. Women who are in their menopause

237.   A person who has debecutis is said to have:
    a. Bedsore or skin ulcer
    b. Dentures
    c. Limp joints and fungus

238.   State which is the best ways for a child to inherit healthy eating habits:
    a. Family involvement and easy access to healthy foods
    b. Family involvement and choices to all different types of foods
    c. Schools and friends involvement

239.   Another name for obesity is:
    a. Bulimia
    b. Over-nutrition
    c. Anorexia

240.   A healthy lunch or snack is:
    a. A meal consisting of saturated fat and low-calorie or diet coke
    b. A meal consists of low-fats, oils and sweets, milk or water
    c. A meal consists of low-calorie and low-fat or skim milk

241.   Another name for bleeding is:
    a. Hemorrhage
    b. Stoppage
    c. Tourniquet

242. Rheumatoid arthritis (RA) is:
      a. Joint inflammation
      b. Muscle weakness
      c. Neurological joint weakness

243. Rheumatoid Arthritis (RA) can be diagnosed if you experienced:
      a. Stiffness of joints in the mornings which improved during the day
      b. Pain or tenderness at least in one joint and swelling of at least one joint
      c. All of the above (A & B)

244. Lung cancer, heart disease, emphysema and other respiratory problems are common among:
      a. Smokers
      b. Drug addicts
      c. Obese persons

245. Infants born to smoking mothers tend to be:
      a. Overweight and obese than infants of nonsmokers
      b. Weigh less than infants of nonsmokers
      c. Born premature than infants of nonsmokers

246. An alternative therapy most frequently reported to be helpful for cognitive problem is:
      a. Music therapy
      b. Art therapy
      c. Water therapy

247. T-cells travel the body in both:
      a. Blood and veins
      b. Blood and lymph
      c. Blood and secretion

248. The people who should get the flu vaccine include:
      a. People 65 year of age and older, children ages 6 months to 23 months
      b. Children 2 years and older with chronic lung or heart disorders
      c. All of the above (A & B)

249.   The people who should not take the flu vaccine shots, include anyone
        who is:
        a. Allergic to caffeine, potassium and overweight
        b. Allergic to eggs or has severe reaction to flu shot or fever
        c. Allergic to flax seed oil or on nutritional supplements that contain
            magnesium

250.   Diets rich in fiber and low in fat can help to control symptoms associ-
        ated with:
        a. Diarrhea
        b. Whopping Cough
        c. Menopause

251.   PET scan is used to detect:
        a. Bacterial toxin in the blood stream
        b. Tumors and locate the source of epileptic activity in the brain
        c. Signs of schizophrenia

252.   PET scan is valuable in studying:
        a. Blood flow and cell activity in the damaged heart
        b. Poisons and their antidotes
        c. The end product of microbes that invade the body

253.   A thyroid gland that does not produce enough thyroid hormones is called:
        a. Active thyroid
        b. Semi-active thyroid
        c. Under-active thyroid

254.   Cystic Fibrosis (CF) is a progressive, lifelong condition in which the
        glands that produce mucus, sweat and intestinal secretions do not:
        a. Link the sweat glands
        b. Function properly
        c. Make breathing difficult

255.   The approximate percentage of women who may have lymph-node
        positive breast cancer is:
        a. 10 percent
        b. 20 percent
        c. 30 percent

256.   Prostate cancer death among American affect:
        a. Men, age 35 and older
        b. Women, age 45 and older
        c. Men, age 55 and older

257.   MBI—Mass Body Index best weight should be for:
        a. 5 feet 6 inches—125 lb
        b. 5 feet 6 inches—165 lb
        c. 5 feet 6 inches—195 lb

258.   Digital mammograms can help in:
        a. Early detection of breast cancer
        b. Early detection of prostate cancer
        c. Early detection of oral cancer

259.   The following people need to check for colorectal cancer:
        a. Men
        b. Women
        c. All of the Above (A & B)

260.   What best describes blister:
        a. Pus that forms on top of the skin
        b. Limited collections of fluid under the skin
        c. Large quantity of blood under the skin

261.   Blood consists of many elements of:
        a. Liquid and zinc
        b. Solid and sulfur
        c. Liquid and solid

262.   The adult human body contains:
        a. Between 5 to 6 quarts of blood
        b. Between 8 to 9 quarts of blood
        c. Between 15 to 16 quarts of blood

263.   The blood group that can be given to everyone in an emergency situation is:
    a. Group A blood
    b. Group B blood
    c. Group O blood

264.   Low blood pressure is called:
    a. Hypotension
    b. Photomicrograph
    c. Hypertension

265.   Blood pressure is referred to as:
    a. High and low blood pressure
    b. High, medium and low blood pressure
    c. Extra high and high blood pressure

266.   There are approximately:
    a. 109 bones, 310 muscles, 125 joints in the human body
    b. 150 bones, 390 muscles, 200 joints in the human body
    c. 206 bones, 700 muscles, 250 joints in the human body

267.   The minerals substance deposited to the bones by the body to make them hard is:
    a. Calcium and mineral
    b. Calcium and iron
    c. Calcium and phosphorus

268.   The following people have the longest life spans they get from regular physical exercise, which helps to slow down the aging process:
    a. Sardinia, Costa Rica and Okinawa, Japan
    b. Calgary, Canada and Charlottesville, U.S.A.
    c. Kvarner Bay, Croatia and Denarau Island, Fiji

269.   Prescription drugs have become:
    a. Narcolepsy
    b. An epidemic
    c. A dynamism

270. A whale on the skin is:
    a. An outburst of a whale on the ocean
    b. Clogging of the pores
    c. A swollen, itching area on the skin

271. When someone experiences tachycardia, it means the person has:
    a. Given birth to a premature baby and the baby needs to stay in an incubator
    b. Rapid heart beat, and corresponding fast pulse beat
    c. Weakness in the joints, especially the fingers

272. Any tumor or new growth that includes embryonic tissue is called:
    a. Teratoma
    b. Tonsils
    c. Thorax

273. The art of science for healing the sick is called:
    a. Therapeutics
    b. Excrement
    c. Tympanitis

274. The acronym Q.I.D. on a prescription means:
    a. Four times a day
    b. Quit intake during the day
    c. Question and information defense

275. Another name for pile is:
    a. Oxidizer
    b. Hemorrhoids
    c. Influenza

276. Piles or hemorrhoids are swollen or varicose veins either outside, inside or across the wall of the:
    a. Armpit
    b. Anus
    c. Vagina

277.   Pityriasis is a:
    a. Skin symptom marked by the presence of hives
    b. Arthritis of the joints experienced by older people
    c. Skin disease marked by the presence of scales or flakes

278.   Pneumonia is an inflammation of the:
    a. Lungs
    b. Skull
    c. Stomach

279.   The answer that best describe who gets pneumonia is:
    a. No one is immune
    b. Younger children, three months to eighteen months
    c. Older people, over 65 years old

280.   Hypostatic pneumonia usually occurring in:
    a. Younger children, usually those of weaker immune system
    b. Elderly, bed-ridden patients
    c. Overweight people

281.   Lipoid pneumonia usually occurring in:
    a. Elderly
    b. Adults
    c. Young children

282.   People who get pneumonia, the death rate is:
    a. Higher in the winter
    b. Lower in the winter
    c. Higher in the summer

283.   Pneumonia usually begins:
    a. With a cough followed by running nose often experienced in colder climates
    b. Following a neglected cold or other conditions that lowers body resistance
    c. An allergy and which turns into a cold

284. Someone suspected of gas poisoning and is unconscious, you must:
    a. Call emergency immediately
    b. Be given water to drink immediately
    c. Move the person away from the gas area and wait for recovery

285. A good way to slow down and charm your stress is to:
    a. Have a few cups of coffee every day
    b. Meditate—give yourself at least 2 to 5 minutes of silence every day
    c. Drink a couple of Brandy or whiskey at night before going to bed

286. Gastric acidity is sometimes increased by:
    a. Tonsillitis
    b. Walking
    c. Smoking

287. The number of kids diagnosed with Autism in America is:
    a. One in 100,000
    b. One in 1,200
    c. One in 150

288. Caesarean section is:
    a. Aligning the section of the womb to accommodate new birth
    b. Delivery of an infant through an incision in the abdominal wall of the uterus
    c. Opening between the throat and the stomach walls

289. Cells found in the human body are:
    a. Epithelial cells and nerve cells
    b. Connective tissue cells and blood cells, muscle cells and sex cells
    c. All of the above (A & B)

290. Another name for cerumen is:
    a. Earwax
    b. Vertebrae
    c. Eye trouble

291.   The Cervix is the:
        a. Inside of the womb
        b. Neck of the womb
        c. Male sex organ

292.   Another name for 'change of life' is:
        a. Old age
        b. Toddler
        c. Menopause

293.   Chicken pox is:
        a. Not a contagious disease
        b. A contagious disease, especially in its early stages
        c. A contagious disease, especially in the late stages of outbreak

294.   Childbirth is a:
        a. Natural and normal process
        b. Unnatural and normal process
        c. Abnormal and unusual process

295.   Following delivery (after childbirth), the mother usually:
        a. Walk
        b. Sleep
        c. Shower

296.   Three factors that increase your risk of experiencing heart attack, angina or a stroke is:
        a. Lack of exercise, low immune system and overweight
        b. Low blood pressure, smoking and low cholesterol
        c. High blood pressure, smoking and high cholesterol

297.   To get the chill is:
        a. A sudden feeling of being warm
        b. A sudden feeling of being hot
        c. A sudden feeling of being cold

298. Chill is accompanied by:
   a. Shivering and chattering of teeth
   b. Shivering and shaking of the knees
   c. Shivering and laughing

299. A chiropodist is:
   a. A doctor who treats back pains
   b. A foot specialist who treats minor ailments of the feet
   c. An eye specialist who operates on major eye surgery

300. Chloroform is:
   a. An effective painkiller
   b. An inflammation in the thyroid
   c. A weak form of painkiller given after childbirth

301. Circumcision is:
   a. Cutting away the foreskin of the penis
   b. Cutting away the foreskin of the vagina
   c. Sterilizing the foreskin of the penis

302. For someone to feel claustrophobic, it means the person has:
   a. Near sightedness
   b. Abnormal fear of height over six feet or more
   c. Abnormal fear of being in a closed space

303. Conception is:
   a. Misconception of the ovum by the sperm
   b. Fertilization of the fetus by the sperm
   c. Fertilization of the ovum by the sperm

304. Concussion of the brain is a bruise of the brain, the result of:
   a. A blow to the head, fall or other violence to the head
   b. A fall or blow to the face
   c. Hit in the head by a soft object

305. The best age for girls to begin visiting a gynecologist is:
   a. Age nine
   b. Age thirteen
   c. Age eighteen

306.   In mild cases of concussion, one may experience:
        a. Slight dizziness and headache
        b. Neck pain
        c. A and B

307.   Congenital heart disease is any heart disease present at:
        a. Conception
        b. Birth
        c. Growth

308.   To defecate is to:
        a. Move the bowels or discharge feces
        b. Decay in the spinal cord nerves
        c. All of the above (A & B)

309.   Dehydration is the condition that results when:
        a. An excessive or abnormal amount of water is removed from the body
        b. An excessive or abnormal amount of water is placed in the body
        c. Someone does not intake eight glasses of water in a day

310.   A newborn baby is supported for:
        a. The first one-month
        b. The first two months
        c. The first three months

311.   The number of breaths given at the beginning of CPR is:
        a. One breath
        b. Two breaths
        c. Five breathes

312.   Dehydration may result from extreme:
        a. Perspiration, repeated vomiting, urination or diarrhea
        b. Vomiting and diarrhea
        c. Lack of eating, drinking, diarrhea and vomiting

313.   A balanced diet contains six essentials of human nutrition. They are:
        a. Proteins, carbohydrates, fats, vitamins, minerals and water
        b. Proteins, carbohydrates, calcium, minerals, magnesium and milk
        c. Carbohydrates, calcium, vitamins, minerals, phosphorus and water

314.   Dizziness is a:
        a. Common symptom of alertness during a sudden fright
        b. Common symptom of headache pains
        c. Common symptom of a disease or body disturbance

315.   The scanning procedure that uses radio waves emitted in a powerful
        magnetic field to create detail images of organs and other soft tissue of
        the internal structures is called a:
        a. PET scan
        b. MRI
        c. Biopsy

316.   Disorientation is a:
        a. State of mental confusion and recognition
        b. State of mental alertness and understanding
        c. State of being able to lie still for short periods

317.   Your teeth are covered with a sticky, colorless film of bacteria called:
        a. Enamel
        b. Plaque
        c. Bleaching

318.   The three main parts of the human ear are:
        a. The outer, middle ear and inner ear
        b. The outer, inner and ear drum
        c. The outer, canal and inner ear

319.   The function of the ear is to provide:
        a. The sense of hearing, to maintain our equilibrium
        b. To maintain a sense of balance
        c. All of the above (A & B)

320.   The most essential part of the hearing apparatus is:
        a. The outer ear
        b. The oval ear
        c. The inner ear

321.   Eczema is a:
    a. Skin disease or disorder
    b. Skin disease rashes
    c. Skin rashes or disease

322.   Epilepsy is a condition characterized by:
    a. Sudden disturbances of the brain function
    b. Temporarily impairment of consciousness
    c. All of the above (A & B)

323.   Itching is a combination of the:
    a. Sense of itching and touching
    b. Sense of touch and skin inflammation
    c. Sense of touch and pain

324.   Jaundice is a serious symptom of disease that causes the:
    a. Skin, the whites of the eyes and mucous membranes to turn yellow
    b. Whites of the eyes to turn yellow
    c. Whites of the eyes and mucous membranes to turn yellowish

325.   Joints dislocations occur most commonly at the:
    a. Knee, shoulder and elbow joints
    b. Neck, shoulder, elbow, palm and toes
    c. Shoulder, elbow and in the fingers and toes

326.   How do you catch a cold?
    a. From someone who has a cold
    b. From going outside in the cold without proper attire
    c. From going in a hot to cold climate

327.   Exhaustion is the state of being:
    a. Exhilarated and relaxed
    b. Worn out with extreme fatigue
    c. Refreshed and feeling relieved

328.   Enuresis or bed-wetting is usually due to a:
    a. Physical factors
    b. Emotional factors
    c. Psychological factors

329.   Epidemic is the:
a. Skin disease affecting a great number of people in a community
b. Widespread attack of a particular disease in a community
c. A drug used to control a widespread of particular disease in a community

330.   Embryo is a:
a. Fertilized seed or egg is in the process of growing
b. Living organism in its earliest stages
c. All of the above (A and B)

331.   How much exercise one should take, depends on:
a. Age, sex and physical condition
b. How long you have been exercising in the past
c. Body size and age

332.   The most common cause of obstructed airway in adults is:
a. Cookies
b. Smoking
c. Meats

333.   Diaper rash is a skin ailment found:
a. Under the armpit of infants and older adults
b. Around the crease of the neck of smaller children
c. Buttocks and genitals of infants and some bedridden adults

334.   If someone has a diarrhea, it usually means the person is having:
a. Low frequency of stool and lots of sweating
b. Frequent and excessive bowel movement
c. Hard pieces of stool in a regular bowel movement

335.   Diastole is the:
a. Flowing of blood to the bloodstreams
b. Blood pressure equipment
c. Resting stage of the heart between beats

336.　An extrovert is a:
　　　a. Personality type that is outwardly happy and playful
　　　b. Personality type that is also referred to as introvert
　　　c. Personality type that turns to the outside world

337.　Glaucoma is a:
　　　a. Minor eye disease
　　　b. Serious eye disease
　　　c. Rare blood disease

338.　Fainting is a result of a:
　　　a. Diminished supply of blood to the brain
　　　b. Diminished supply of blood to the veins
　　　c. Increase supply of blood to the brain

339.　The human foot is designed and engineered for:
　　　a. Forward locomotion
　　　b. Backward locomotion
　　　c. Rearward movement

340　Poor posture in standing or walking can cause:
　　　a. Blisters
　　　b. Flat foot
　　　c. Arch weakness

341　Gallstones—who is are affected more:
　　　a. Twice as frequently as men
　　　b. Women, five times as frequently as men
　　　c. Twenty-five times as frequently as men

342.　Gall-bladder attacks usually come in:
　　　a. Young age
　　　b. Middle age
　　　c. Old age

343.　A heart attack is eminent:
　　　a. When a coronary artery is closed up
　　　b. When a coronary artery is opened up
　　　c. When someone who is overweight and exercise

344.   Hepatitis is an inflammation of the:
a. Stomach
b. Mouth
c. Liver

345.   Illusion is compared with:
a. Ongoing pain
b. Delusion and hallucination
c. Semi consciousness and hallucination

346.   The immune system has three main functions:
a. To protect, to evolve and to distinguish
c. To protect, to establish and to guide
c. To protect, to maintain and to serve

347.   The American National Multiple Sclerosis (MS) Society estimates that some:
a. 75,000 Americans have MS
b. 400,000 American have MS
c. 750,000 Americans have MS

348.   Immunization is to provide:
a. Immunity against infectious diseases by injections
b. Susceptibility to infectious diseases by injections
c. Counteraction against polio and smallpox diseases

349.   Herpes is a:
a. Virus infection in which blisters develop on the skin
b. Virus infection in which the whole body is affected by hives
c. Abnormal growth of the hipbone

350.   Another name for hypertension is:
a. Hypotension or "the no symptom killer"
b. High blood pressure or "the silent killer"
c. Low blood pressure or "postmenopausal"

351. Another name for hypotension is:
a. Hypertension
b. High blood pressure
c. Low blood pressure

352. Infection is the:
a. Entry, presence and multiplication of disease-producing microbes in the body
b. Presence and multiplication of disease-producing microbes in the human body
c. None of the above

353. Inflammation is the reaction of:
a. Active body tissue when exposed and become infected
b. Body tissue to injury, whether by infection or trauma
c. Centralized body tissue to injury, either external or internal organs

354. Heredity is:
a. The study between animals and people
b. The study of the environment, people and animals
c. The likeness between parents and children

355. Trouble in the joints is evidenced by:
a. Pain, stiffness, swelling, redness, heat and infection
b. Pain, stiffness, swelling, redness, heat and loss of motion
c. Pain, stiffness, swelling, infection, injury and nervous system

356. The course of the influenza disease may run from:
a. Two days to many weeks
b. Seven days to twenty weeks
c. Only for a short time, but not more than a week

357 An inhaler is:
a. An anesthetic or other drugs administered by breathing into the mouth
b. An injection that is usually administered by a breathing apparatus
c. An apparatus for breathing in volatile drugs in vapor state

358. If a doctor says that a patient is inoperable it usually means that it is:
a. Too soon for operation, especially in cancer
b. Too late for operation, especially in cancer
c. Too late for operation, especially in childbirth

359. Select the correct group with all insects in it:
a. Mosquitoes, ticks, lice, hedgehog and itch mites
b. Mosquitoes, fleas, lice, spiders and benzyl benzoate
c. Mosquitoes, ticks, lice, fleas, itch mites and bedbugs

360. Intelligence is the ability of a human being to:
a. Unscrambled codes and put them into understandable words
b. Understand and comprehend what is sensed
c. Make the prerequisite of jumble words be understood

361. Intelligence is measured by terms of:
a. Intelligence Quotient (I.Q.)
b. Mental age and intelligence quotient (I.Q.)
c. Mental deficiency and intelligence quotient (I.Q.)

362. Chronic diarrhea may be a symptom of:
a. Colon cancer
b. Breast cancer
c. Prostate cancer

363. The symptom of colon cancer include:
a. Stomach and discomfort in the breast
b. Mouth and changes in bowel habits
c. Stomach and changes in bowel habits

364. Malignant is medical terminology refers primary to:
a. Bowel
b. Spleen
c. Cancer

365. Measles is:
a. An infectious disease, usually of childhood
b. An acute, infectious disease, usually of childhood
c. A mild, non-infectious disease, usually of childhood

366.   Menstruation known as monthly period, is the:
        a. Constant discharge of blood from the vagina
        b. Periodic discharge of blood from the vagina
        c. Constant discharge of sperm from the penis

367.   Parkinson's disease is known as:
        a. Lymph nodes
        b. Schizophrenia
        c. Shaking palsy

368.   The teenage time of life when the sex organs develop is called:
        a. Puberty
        b. Adult
        c. Menopause

369.   Shingle is:
        a. A virus infection
        b. A benign cancer
        c. A rush in blood pressure following a fall

370.   Juvenile Rheumatoid Arthritis is a:
        a. Pain disease in children's body
        b. Chronic inflammatory disease in children's joints
        c. Chronic inflammatory disease found in young adult's joints

371.   Skin rash is identifiable with:
        a. Cracking
        b. Dryness
        c. Hitching

372.   Small pox vaccination is carried out at:
        a. Three to six months old
        b. Three to twelve months old
        c. Twelve to twenty-four months old

373. The persons that have a higher rate of lung cancer, heart disease, emphysema and other respiratory problems are:
   a. Vegetarian
   b. Dieters
   c. Smokers

374. Pregnancy begins with conception and ends with:
   a. A boy
   b. Childbirth
   c. A girl

375. Exercise strengthens the … and builds bone mass and muscle mass:
   a. Digestive system
   b. Lungs and digestive systems
   c. Heart and lung muscles

376. PSA is the acronym for:
   a. Prostate Specific Antigen
   b. Prostate Sterilization Arteriole
   c. Prostate Specific Audiometer

377. It is reported that walking reduces:
   a. Flat feet
   b. Energy level
   c. Breast cancer

378. A phobia is:
   a. Fear of height
   b. Fear of height or darkness
   c. Fear of an object, circumstance or situation

379. Wheezing is associated with:
   a. Sinus
   b. Snoring
   c. Breathing

380.   During times of illness, the body's natural defenses against my be:
       a. Jolted
       b. Weakened
       c. Communized

381.   The vitamin that helps to preserve the integrity of the skin, making it
       somewhat more resistant to infection is:
       a. Vitamin A
       b. Vitamin B
       c. Vitamin C

382.   Liver, milk, egg yolk, many green and yellow vegetables, where it exist
       as carotene you will find:
       a. Vitamin A
       b. Vitamin B
       c. Vitamin C

383.   A back massage does what:
       a. Makes you feel good
       b. Stresses the muscles and makes the person sleeps
       c. Relaxes muscles and stimulates circulation

384.   The daily-recommended servings of breads, cereals, rice and pasta are:
       a. Three to six
       b. Five to twelve
       c. Seven to sixteen

385.   They daily servings of the meat groups recommended are:
       a. One only
       b. Two to three
       c. Four to five

386.   AIDS is usually spread by contact with:
       a. Saliva
       b. Sharing same cup
       c. Infected blood

387. A person with Down syndrome always has:
      a. Some degree of mental retardation
      b. Some degree of spinal injuries
      c. Some degree of swelling in the brain

388. Autism begins:
      a. At fertilization
      b. Early childhood
      c. Late childhood

389. Urine is formed in the:
      a. Bowel
      b. Kidneys
      c. Intestines

390. Solid foods are usually given to a baby during the:
      a. Fifth or sixth month
      b. Eight or nine month
      c. Tenth or eleventh month

391. Alcohol affects the:
      a. Blood stream
      b. Nervous systems
      c. Nerve cell of the brain

392. Alcohol when taken in small amounts:
      a. Impairs vision
      b. Is good for the body
      c. Impairs judgment and coordination

393. The parts of the body in which allergy reactions show up are:
      a. Skin, ear, eye, teeth and tongue
      b. Skin, digestive system, nose and bronchial tree
      c. Bowel, skin, nose and uterus

394. Oral cancer usually affects:
      a. Younger men, but can develop in anyone
      b. Older men, but can develop in anyone
      c. Younger women, but can develop in anyone

395.   Oral cancer is a sore or lump on the lip or in the:
    a. Mouth or throat
    b. Mouth or lip
    c. Gum and lip

396.   Older persons should avoid dry foods because of:
    a. Gum problems
    b. Decrease in saliva
    c. Teeth and throat is smaller

397.   VD known as venereal disease is a:
    a. Disease spread by kissing
    b. Symptom spread by body-to-body contact
    c. Disease spread by sexual intercourse

398.   The last teeth to erupt are the:
    a. Wisdom teeth or third molars
    b. Wisdom teeth or periodontal membrane
    c. Wisdom teeth or first molars

399.   Women should do breasts self-examinations:
    a. Once a day
    b. Once a month
    c. Once a year

400.   The flu is mostly common in the fall and winter. The best answer that
        describes the flu is:
    a. Relatively non-existence in the summer months
    b. Only attacks older people
    c. Highly contagious

SECTION V

This is the Advanced Section, questions 401 through to 800. Good luck!

ADVANCED QUESTIONS

401. After menopause, your risk of developing hypertension is likely to:
    a. Decrease significantly
    b. Increase significantly
    c. Have no significant change

402. Another name for spontaneous abortion is:
    a. Miscarriage
    b. Illegal abortion
    c. Delinquent abortion

403. Arterigram/angiogram test is used to:
    a. Examine a patient's arteries
    b. Examine a patient's blood
    c. Examine a patient's temperature

404. Open and closed biopsies require:
    a. Immobilizing
    b. Closing
    c. Incisions

405. Reduced blood supply to the brain can result in:
    a. Improved memory
    b. Confession and drowsiness
    c. Confusion and dizziness

406.   Fatigue is frustrating in individuals with MS. It can last for only a short
        period of time or for years, and:
        a. It can be mild or completely debilitating
        b. It can be mild and bearable
        c. It can be mild or manageable

407.   Diagnosis of fatigue in people living with MS is done by:
        a. Sex, age, diet and where you live
        b. Your personal health, family history, age and environment
        c. Personal health, family history, a physical examination and labora-
           tory tests

408.   The people who are at risk of having uterine cancer are:
        a. Women who are obese, infertile or have menstrual problems
        b. Men who are obese, suffers a heart attack or experienced thyroid
           problems
        c. All of the above (A & B)

409.   Albumin is a protein substance found in:
        a. Animal tissues only
        b. Human tissues only
        c. All of the above (A & B)

410.   Hemoglobin is the substance in the red blood cells that carries:
        a. Oxygen and gives blood its color
        b. Food to the intestines and gives blood its color
        c. White blood cells and turns blood to red blood cells

411.   Good nutrition is needed for:
        a. Growth, healing and maintaining body functions
        b. Growing and good bones
        c. Growth, body weight and body functions

412.   Another term to refer to amenorrhea is:
        a. Poor vision
        b. The morning after pill
        c. Absence of menstruation

413.   Some of the amino acids found in food or as medicine are:
    a. Asparagines and tryptophan
    b. Glycine, Glutamic acid and histidine
    c. All of the above (A & B)

414.   Anemia is:
    a. An increase in the number of circulating red blood cells
    b. A decrease in the number of circulating white blood cells
    c. A decrease in the number of circulating red blood cells

415.   Anemia is caused by:
    a. A lack of iron in the diet
    b. An increase of too much iron in the diet
    c. The white blood cells colliding with the red blood cells

416.   When someone has anemia it means there is:
    a. An increase in the number of circulating red blood cell
    b. A decrease in the number of circulating red blood cell
    c. A decrease in iron deficiency

417.   Angina is:
    a. A sensation occurring before death
    b. Any repeated, suffocating pain or the disease that caused it
    c. An important substance produced in the body that protects it from
        disease

418.   Antiseptics are usually used in or on human body to:
    a. Inhibit the growth of disease-producing micro-organisms
    b. Increase the growth of disease-producing microorganisms
    c. Speed up the growth of disease-producing microorganisms

419.   Excessive urine many depict:
    a. Parkinson disease
    b. Diabetes
    c. Colon cancer

420.   Arachnophism is related to:
    a. Poisoning by spider bite
    b. Poisoning by mosquito bite
    c. Too little of vitamin in the diet

421.   Types of arthritis are:
    a. Rheumatoid and degenerative arthritis
    b. Rheumatoid and salicylates arthritis
    c. Degenerative and Endocrine arthritis

422.   Aspermia relates to:
    a. The performance of artificial respiration
    b. The absence of sperm in semen
    c. Drugs given to relief nasal pain

423.   Atelectasis refers to:
    a. Collapse of the lung
    b. Fatty deposits on the heart
    c. Standard measurement of atomic energy

424.   Alcohol and narcotics affect oxygen flow because they:
    a. Slows down thinking in the brain
    b. Increases too much blood flow to the brain
    c. Depresses the brain

425.   Auricular fibrillation is a form of:
    a. Estrogen
    b. Heart disease
    c. Swollen in the arteries

426.   Cystic Fibrosis causes:
    a. No harm to the digestive system or any difficulty with breathing
    b. Poor digestion, and males with this disease are usually fertile
    c. Poor digestion, and males with this disease are usually infertile

427.   Chronic barbiturates poisoning produces:
    a. Large opening to the airway and heavy blood flow to the veins
    b. Dullness of memory, loss of memory and hallucinations
    c. Cirrhosis and jaundice supply

428. Biopsy is an important technique of diagnosis in:
a. Birth control
b. An infectious disease of the throat
c. Suspected cancer

429. Bladder is parts of the:
a. Urinary system that stores and release urine
b. Hemoglobin found in the urine
c. Human heart that flows the blood to the spine

430. It is recommended that women should get their first bone density scan by:
a. Age 45
b. Age 75
c. Age 80

431. A person with head or spinal cord injuries require:
a. Bed rest
b. Rehabilitation
c. Exercises

432. Hoarseness is the result of:
a. Shouting and loud noise experienced
b. Cancer in the throat
c. Inflammation or swelling of the vocal cords

433. Abnormal bleeding may indicate a:
a. Platelet or clotting factor abnormality
b. Excess blood found on the sheets
c. Wound that is not healing

434. Excessive blood loss often results of anemia. Indicate present sites of unusual bleeding:
a. Nosebleeds and bleeding from the gum
b. Black, tarry stools
c. All of the above (A & B)

435.   Someone can get fever blister of the lips from:
    a. Sun burns
    b. Mosquito, dog bites, contact with poison ivy
    c. Burns and Spanish fly; from contact with poison ivy

436.   Explain where water blisters are formed:
    a. A water blister involves the upper layer of the skin
    b. A water blister involves the lower layer of the skin
    c. A water blister involves both the upper and lower of the skin

437.   Choose the answer that best describes blood:
    a. The red and white blood cells of the organ
    b. The red fluid that circulates throughout the body via the blood vessels
    c. The red fluid that stops in between heartbeats and the blood vessels

438.   Name the three different types of blood cells:
    a. Red, green and orange blood cells
    b. Blood platelets and white blood cells
    c. Red and white blood cells; blood platelets

439.   Another name for red blood cells:
    a. Lymphocytes
    b. Erythrocytes
    c. Bilateral

440.   If you experience persistent gastrointestinal systems movement, doctors can use a … to determine the source of the problems:
    a. Colostomy
    b. Stenosis
    c. Colonoscopy

441.   Blood pressure is the force wielded by the blood beating against the:
    a. Mouth of the heart
    b. Artery walls
    c. Blood vessels

442.   Before a blood transfusion if given, the blood of:
a. One recipient must be matched
b. One donor must be typed and matched
c. Both recipient and donor must be typed and matched

443.   The blood vessels consist of:
a. Veins that carry the blood to the entire body
b. Tubes of varying sizes that carry blood throughout the body to and from the heart
c. Veins from small to large carrying the blood from the brain to the stomach

444.   The musculoskeletal system is made up of:
a. Cartilage, joints and muscles
b. Muscles, joints and ligaments
c. Muscles and cartilage

445.   Osteomyelitis (bone disease) is:
a. Inflammation of the bone due to fractured bone disease
b. Inflammation of the central cavity
c. Inflammation of the bone and central cavity

446.   Multiple sclerosis attacks and destroys myelin:
a. The insulation that protects nerve fibers (axons)
b. The membranes covering the brain
c. The congenital malformations

447.   Syphilis and tuberculosis (bone disease) can:
a. Damage the nervous systems
b. Damage the cornea
c. Damage the bones

448.   Congenital malformations of the bones are found in:
a. Clubfoot and dislocations of the hip and other joints
b. The hip, finger and toes
c. Gaul bladder

449.   Botulism is a:
     a. Concussion received from a fall
     b. A severe and often fatal form of food poisoning
     c. A rare form of mild food poisoning

450.   The human brain consists of:
     a. Skull, spinal cord, cannabis and hypothalamus
     b. Cardiac, vertebra, brain stem, cranial nerve and cortex
     c. Skull, cerebrum, thalamus, upper spinal cord and cerebellum

451.   A person who has Parkinson's disease will show:
     a. Signs of slow movements
     b. Signs and symptoms of still muscles
     c. All of the above (A & B)

452.   Cerebral hemorrhage bleeding is caused by:
     a. The breaking of a blood vessel in the brain
     b. The breaking of a vein in the brain
     c. The opening of the brain that surrounds the skull

453.   Brain tumor is a:
     a. Pressure on the skull of the brain membrane
     b. Growth of new and unwanted tissue in the brain
     c. Growth and abscess in the brain

454.   Cancer originating in the breast frequently spread to the:
     a. Neck, nose, large intestine and stomach
     b. Breast and stomach
     c. Prostate gland, kidney and stomach

455.   The heart of an average adult beats approximately:
     a. 45 times per minute
     b. 72 times per minute
     c. 120 times per minute

456.   To get cachexia is:
     a. Extreme weight loss and weakness as a result of serious diseases
     b. Extreme weight gain and laziness as a result of not exercising
     c. An extreme cough that brings on hoarseness

457.   Caduceus is a:
       a. Weakness in the bowel
       b. Common symbol of medicine
       c. Redness in the corner of the eye

458.   Calcification is the deposit of:
       a. Callus to the hands and feet
       b. Steroids to nervous systems
       c. Calcium into the body tissues

459.   Another name for calculus is:
       a. Calcium or uterus
       b. Calcium or rock stone
       c. Gallstone or kidney stone

460.   Select the one that best describes callus:
       a. Soften and moistures the skin
       b. Hardened and thickened skin
       c. Produced growth hormones

461.   Cancer cells can start in:
       a. Any part of the body, but some sites are more favored
       b. Stomach, breast or throat first
       c. Blood streams and spreads to other parts of the body

462.   Cancer cells are:
       a. Same as ordinary cells
       b. Same as all the cells in the body
       c. Different from ordinary cells

463.   Breast cancer examination should be done by:
       a. Monthly examination of the breast; in front of a mirror
       b. Every morning and night while lying in bed
       c. Every six months by a doctor of sphygmomanometer

464.   Heart disease and stroke account for:
       a. 25 percent of deaths in people with diabetes
       b. 65 percent of deaths in people with diabetes
       c. 75 percent of deaths in people with diabetes

465.   The major risk factor of colorectal cancer is:
        a. Sexual orientation
        b. Weight
        c. Age

466.   Causalgia is a:
        a. Bone that extends from the neck to abdomen
        b. Burning pain sensation
        c. Stimulant within the organ systems

467.   A person with osteoporosis is at risk for:
        a. Fractures
        b. Spinal cord injuries
        c. Stiff muscles

468.   Cerebral hemorrhage is:
        a. Heavy bleeding
        b. Bleeding in the brain; resulting in stroke
        c. Bleeding in the stomach and comes out the rectum

469.   Cerebral Palsy is:
        a. Animal disabilities; is often never live past three months
        b. Infant disabilities; is only experienced inside the womb
        c. Childhood disabilities; is lack of muscular control

470.   Cerebral Palsy arises from:
        a. Cord wrapped around baby's neck during birth
        b. Brain damage before, during or soon after birth
        c. Weakness in the joints

471.   Cerebrum is the:
        a. Small, main lower thinking part of the brain
        b. Small, main upper part of the brain
        c. Large, main, upper thinking part of the brain

472.   Cheilitis is:
        a. Inflammation of the joints and sometimes the fingers
        b. Inflammation of the lips and sometimes corner of the mouth
        c. Inflammation of the veins carrying the blood to the heart

473.   Cheilitis is caused by:
    a. Sunburn, lipstick and chemical irritants
    b. Cystic fibrosis, chemical irritants and allergy
    c. All of the above

474.   Someone can get chilblain in:
    a. Hot weather
    b. Cold weather
    c. After you get sunburn

475.   To protect against chilblain, you need proper protection for the:
    a. Eyelids, scalp and mouth
    b. Finger and toes
    c. Toes; fingers and ears

476.   Child birthing is divided into three stages. Put them in correct order:
    a. Labor pain, full dilation; birth to expulsion of the afterbirth
    b. Full dilation, labor pain; birth to expulsion of the afterbirth
    c. Labor pain, birth; full dilation to expulsion of the afterbirth

477.   Childbirth labor pain begins in the:
    a. Stomach and progress to the vaginal area
    b. Breasts and progress to the stomach
    c. Small of back and progress to the abdomen

478.   If a child becomes withdrawn it is a sign that:
    a. The child is difficult
    b. The child maybe abused
    c. The child is seeking attention

479.   With the guidance of a babysitter, a child can watch the following TV programs:
    a. A pornography movie and gun-fighting movie
    b. A movie where the swear words are blocked out
    c. None of the above

480.   A person with sudden cardiac arrest is:
        a. Sudden stopping of the heart and breathing
        b. Gradually slow breathing of the heart and slow pulse
        c. Sudden slow breathing of the heart and stopping

481.   The nanny puts the baby in the crib to sleep, and expects the baby to
        sleep for at least an hour before the baby wakes up. The nanny has time
        to:
        a. To walk to the corner store to get milk, which would take approxi-
           mately ten minutes
        b. To jog around the block for 5 minutes or to the corner store, which
           takes 2 minutes
        c. None of the above

482.   The baby is choking an adult needs to get the food out:
        a. Hold the baby upside down and shake gently
        b. Dislodge with finger and call emergency
        c. All of the above (A & B)

483.   Cholecystectomy is:
        a. Surgical removal of the gall bladder
        b. Non-surgical removal of the gall bladder
        c. Inflammation of the gall bladder

484.   Cholecystitis is:
        a. Non-surgical treatment of the gall bladder
        b. Inflammation of the gall bladder
        b. Surgical removal of the gall bladder

485.   Cholesterol is:
        a. A fatlike substance found in all animal fats and oils
        b. Found in many other tissues of the human body
        c. All of the above (A and B)

486.   Chorioretinitis is:
        a. Bowel disease
        b. An eye disease
        c. An ear disease

487. The most common methods to determine that a person is chocking is:
    a. Clutching the throat
    b. Loud coughing sound
    c. Pointing at the stomach

488. Cicatrix is a:
    a. Bowel movement, caused by not been able to control
    b. Scar tissue, the flesh that forms when a wound heals
    c. Blood clot or the mass that forms when blood clots

489. Clitoris is the:
    a. Male sex organ
    b. Human and animal sex organs
    c. Female sex organ

490. Clubfoot is:
    a. A large bump on the foot of a small child
    b. A deformity of the foot twisted at the ankle
    c. A deformity of the foot with a bump and patch at the ankle

491. Cocaine is a:
    a. Narcotic drug obtained from coca leaves
    b. Tonic drug obtained from coca leaves
    c. Blood clotting narcotic drug obtained from coca leaves

492. Indicate which of the following describes codcine:
    a. Codeine is a narcotic drug which is related to morphine
    b. Codeine relates to cramps
    c. Codeine is all of the above

493. Colitis is also known as:
    a. Regular bowel movement
    b. Sore bowel
    c. Sore rectum

494. Colitis is caused by:
    a. The red fluid that circulates in the blood cell
    b. The red blood cells known as erythrocytes
    c. Inflammation and visible changes in the bowel

495.   Colon also known as the large intestine:
        a. Extends from the cecum to the rectum
        b. Extends from the cecum to the vagina
        c. Extends from the cecum to the penis

496.   Colostomy is a surgical operation in which:
        a. The colon is brought to form a permanent opening in the abdomen
        b. The colon is brought to form a temporary opening in the abdomen
        c. The colon is brought to replace the temporary opening in the abdomen

497.   The Colostomy bag is worn to receive:
        a. Urine
        b. Blood samples
        c. Bowel movement

498.   In severe or more serious cases of concussion, one may experience:
        a. Upset stomach, heartburn and giddiness
        b. Neck pain, strong pulse, heavy breathing and headache
        c. Nausea and vomiting, weak pulse and slow breathing

499.   Congestion is the accumulation of blood in any part of the body or:
        a. Inflammation of the body tissue
        b. Blockage of the artery
        c. Mucous secretion in the lungs

500.   Constipation is the:
        a. Retention of body fluids in the bowel
        b. Spasms of the bowel
        c. Retention of feces or inability to have a bowel movement

501.   Constipation is a:
        a. Disease of the uterus and hardening of blood vessels
        b. Symptom of hardening of stool in the bowel; or other bowel problems
        c. Frequent bowel movement

502.   Another name for 'consumption' is:
        a. Cramps
        b. Tuberculosis
        c. Hepatitis C

503.   Cornea is the:
    a. Transparent part of the brain
    b. Muscular fatigue of the eyes
    c. Transparent front membrane of the eyes

504.   Someone who has a coryza, it means that the person has:
    a. Running eyes, indicating tiredness
    b. The appearance of the skin tone
    c. Running nose, indicating an acute head cold

505.   To have a cough is a sign that something is wrong in the:
    a. Throat or lungs
    b. Mouth or throat
    c. Bowel or stomach

506.   The principal cause of death in the 1900's, in order, was:
    a. Diarrhea, tuberculosis, diseases and malformations of infants
    b. Heart disease, diarrhea, pneumonia and stroke
    c. Tuberculosis, pneumonia, diarrhea and heart disease

507.   The principal cause of death in America in the 2000's, in order, were:
    a. Heart disease, cancer, stroke and accidents
    b. Accidents, pneumonia, cancer and tuberculosis
    c. Hepatitis C, cancer, tuberculosis and meningitis

508.   Decalcification is the disappearance of:
    a. Calcium from the blood stream, thinning the blood
    b. Calcium from the bones or teeth, strengthening them
    c. Calcium from the bones or teeth, weakening them

509.   Delirium is the state of:
    a. Incoherent, excitement and restlessness
    b. Restlessness, vomiting and nausea
    c. None of the above

510.   A person with delusion is a:
    a. Happy countenance and is usually free from stress
    b. False belief or irrational idea that a mentally person has
    c. Disease of the nervous system that happens to older people

511.   Demography relates to:
    a. Age, sex, finance, nationality and prestige
    b. Age, race, school, and living conditions
    c. Age, sex, race, place of birth and occupation

512.   To prevent cavities you should visit the dentist at least:
    a. Once every two months
    b. Once every six months
    c. Once a year

513.   Depression is a form of:
    c. Mental illness
    b. Skin disease
    c. Lung disease

514.   Diabetes mellitus is a diseased state in which the body is:
    a. Unable to manage the flow of blood to the body
    b. Unable to digest sugar and milk in the diet
    c. Unable to manage its food intake properly

515.   As death nears, the last sense to go is:
    a. Seeing
    b. Hearing
    c. Smelling

516.   The signs of death are:
    a. No pulse, respirations or blood pressure
    b. Short breaths, respirations or blood pressure
    c. No pulse, eyes closed or respirations

517.   The most common symptoms of diabetes are:
    a. Loss of sleep, itching and frequent eating habits
    b. Unusual thirst, frequent urination and loss of weight
    c. Lack of bowel movement and loss of sugar in the diet

518.   Diabetes is mostly found among:
    a. Newborns and underweight babies
    b. Men of Indian and Black origins
    c. Middle-aged and overweight or obese individuals

519.   When considering dieting, one should take into consideration:
    a. Balanced diet with extra salt and sugar to promote health
    b. Nutritionally adequate diet to maintain and promote health and vigor
    c. Nutritionally inadequate diet to maintain and promote grow in children

520.   Digestion is the process by which the digestive system:
    a. Takes the food from the mouth into the stomach
    b. Chew the food by mouth and deposits it into the intestines
    c. Breaks down and prepares food substances taken by mouth

521.   Mechanics of digestion is:
    a. Food is chewed in the mouth and swallowed into the intestines
    b. Food is chewed in the mouth and swallowed into the esophagus
    c. Food is chewed in the mouth and swallowed into the stomach

522.   The digestive system, when food is taken in:
    a. Provides the substances necessary for the regulation of body process
    b. Provides the building blocks for cell growth and energy for body function
    c. All of the above (A & B)

523.   Place the digestive system in order:
    a. Mouth, tongue, salivary glands, esophagus and stomach
    b. Mouth, tongue, stomach, uterine wall and intestine
    c. Mouth, tongue, stomach, esophagus and pancreas

524.   The most common herpes virus are:
    a. X factor and Z factor
    b. Type A (causing genital herpes) and type B (causing hexogen)
    c. Type 1 (causing cold sores and blisters) and type 2 (causing genital herpes)

225.   Approximately what number of persons in the United States of America get infections while staying in the hospital?
    a. 100,000
    b. 1 million
    c. 2 million

526.   Deaths resulted from infections caught in a hospital in the U.S each
        year, is approximately:
        a. 25,000
        b. 90,000
        c. 750,000

527.   Commonly known disinfectants are:
        a. Formaldehyde, alcohols and chlorine-releasing compounds
        b. Alcohols, microbes and diplopia
        c. All of the above (A & B)

528.   To prevent hospital infection the staff must:
        a. Wash hands and sterilize instruments
        b. Wear gloves
        c. Don't go to the hospital

529.   When someone has a slipped disk it is a condition in which one of
        these occurred:
        a. Inter-vertebral disks, usually in the lower back, has slipped out of
           place
        b. The result is lower back pain, often severe, bending down often
           becomes exceedingly painful
        c. All of the above (A & B)

530.   Dislocation is referred to as:
        a. Blood flow, usually slow, to the veins
        b. Joints are usually disrupted
        c. Joints are usually in order

531.   Diverticulitis is a:
        a. Disease of the salivary gland
        b. Disease of the large bowel (colon)
        c. Disease of the pancreas

532.   Douche usually refers to:
        a. Irrevocable dizziness caused by over-used douching
        b. Irrigation or cleansing of the vagina
        c. Reliable method of avoiding pregnancy

533.   Drugs sometimes come in contact with the skin, result in which of the following:
a. Corrosives—destroy tissue
b. Disinfectants—destroys microbes
c. All of the above (A & B)

534.   Dysmenorrheal is a:
a. Painful bowel disorder
b. Painful menstruation
c. Painless menstruation

535.   To experience dysphasia it means:
a. Someone is having difficulty swallowing
b. Someone is having difficulty chewing
c. Someone is having a shortness of breath

536.   Dyspnea is referred to:
a. Shortness of breath
b. Heart failure
c. Painful ear pain

537.   Factors that increase the risk of a fall:
a. Weakness, and low blood pressure
b. Poor judgment and foot problems
c. All of the above (A & B)

538.   Trouble in the middle ear is frequently subject to:
a. Infection
b. Wax
c. Deformities

539.   Ecchymosis is a:
a. Black and red spot or other discolored patch on the skin
b. Blue and red spot or other discolored patch on the skin
c. Black and blue spot or other discolored patch on the skin

540.   Ecthyma is a:
        a. Inflammation of the skin; covered by rashes
        b. Skin ailment; red blotches covered with pustules
        c. Foreign bodies with rashes covered with pustules

541.   Electrolysis is a method of:
        a. Implanting hair growth
        b. Promoting hair growth
        c. Removing unwanted hair

542.   Diuretic is anything that promotes:
        a. Excretion of feces
        b. Excretion of urine
        c. Stoppage of urine

543.   Emaciation is:
        a. The wasting away of body tissue
        b. The result of digestive disorders due to skin disorder
        c. None of the above

544.   Embryology is the science of:
        a. Following the development of life after death
        b. Tracing the development of new life from conception to birth
        c. Body cells and circulation in the veins and blood vessels

545.   Empyema is:
        a. A collection of pus in a body cavity
        b. A collection of embryo
        c. A collection of cavity virus

546.   The most common accumulation of pus is found in:
        a. The bone cavity
        b. The chest cavity
        c. The auditory cavity

547.   Encephalitis is:
        a. Inflammation of the stomach
        b. Inflammation of the chest
        c. Inflammation of the brain

548.   Encephalogram is:
        a. An x-ray picture of the brain
        b. An x-ray picture of the mouth
        c. An x-ray picture of the stomach

549.   Another name for enuresis is:
        a. Laziness or sluggishness in waking up
        b. Bed-wetting or involuntary discharge of urine
        c. Walking with a limp on the left foot

550.   Epidemiology is the study of:
        a. Disease as it outbreaks and involves animals and people
        b. Disease investigation
        c. Disease as it spreads and involves large groups of people

551.   Epidermis is the:
        a. Inner layer of the skin
        b. Outer layer of the skin
        c. Pigmentation of the skin

552.   Epidermophytosis is a:
        a. Blood vessel tubes of varying sizes; for example the arteries
        b. Fungus infection of the skin; for example athlete's foot
        c. Ear infection, leading to the brain; for example cerebellum

553.   Genital herpes is a:
        a. Contagious viral infection that spreads through skin and sexual
            contacts
        b. Non contagious viral infection that spreads through skin contact
            and the environment
        c. Non contagious viral outbreak due to stress and other similar
            symptoms

554.   Episiotomy is a minor surgery sometimes performed on:
        a. Men who has testicular cancer
        b. Women during childbirth
        c. Women who have problems with back pain

555.   Episiotomy is a surgical incision to widen the opening:
    a. From the cerumen and present lacerations
    b. From the vagina and present lacerations
    c. From the cervix and present lacerations

556.   Other common herpes infections are:
    a. Chicken pox and shingles
    b. Pollen and colds
    c. Laughing without stopping

557.   Erysipelas is a:
    a. Stomach disease caused by infection of the thinning of the blood
    b. Tumor arising from the epithelium
    c. Skin disease caused by infection with streptococcus germ

558.   Erythroblastosis Fetalis is a:
    a. Blood disorder of older people
    b. Blood disease of animals
    c. Anemia disease of newborn infants

559.   Estrogen is a general name for a large group of closely related:
    a. Male sex hormones
    b. Female sex hormones
    c. Male and female sex organs

560.   A toothache is usually the sign of: other name for euthanasia is:
    a. Ethmoid of the gum
    b. Sinusitis or the need for a new filling
    c. Badly decayed tooth

561.   A regular, appropriate exercise is:
    a. Beneficial for persons with chronic health conditions
    b. Beneficial for children under the age of three
    c. Beneficial for someone who is pregnant and above to give birth

562.   Exercise is especially important in the:
    a. Diagnosing abdominal and menstruation pains
    b. Prevention, diagnosing and rehabilitation of cardiovascular diseases
    c. Prevention, diagnosing and rehabilitation of AIDS patients

563.   Individuals who are asthmatic can:
a. Increase the risks of an attack by exercising
b. Reduce the risks by exercising sparingly before or after the attack
c. Reduce the risks of an attack during by regular exercising

564.   You should conclude your exercise routine with a:
a. Rigid routine, to tone up lax muscles and loosen stiff one
b. Cool down habit, to prevent sudden changes, such as in your heart rate
c. Uncompromising routine to stimulate your heart rate for best results

565.   When you are beginning an exercise program it is best to:
a. Watch what others are doing and follow their routine
b. Only begin with easy ones and stick to them for at least a period of time
c. Use the self-paced approach to determine how you feel and your comfort level

566.   Exercise can:
a. Strengthen your immune system to prevent many ailments
b. Deteriorate your immune system cause more health issues
c. Can shut down your immune system for good

567.   The nervous system does the following:
a. Controls, oblique and coordinates body function
b. Controls, directs and contradicts nervous system
c. Controls, directs and coordinates body function

568.   Expectorant is any remedy that helps a patient:
a. Bring up and spit out excessive secretions from the lungs and windpipe
b. Release the white blood cells into the bloodstreams
c. Ventilate by wearing a feeding tube in the mouth

569.   Mastoiditis is a possible serious infectious complication of:
a. Outer ear
b. Middle ear
c. Inner ear

570.   The human eye is essentially an apparatus for:
        a. Focusing and registering light rays on a vitreous humor, the pupil
        b. Focusing and registering light rays on a light-sensitive membrane, the retina
        c. Focusing and registering light rays on a lens, the cornea

571.   The area of the eye that makes sight possible includes:
        a. The eyeball, optic nerve, cornea and lens
        b. The eyeball, retina, optic nerve, visual center and brain
        c. The eyeball, optic nerve and visual center in the brain

572.   Cataract is a:
        a. Bulging of the eyes out the eye-socket
        b. Clouding of the crystalline lens of the eye or its capsule
        c. An optical distortion of the eye, usually starting in one eye to the next

573.   Pink eye is an epidemic form of conjunctivitis, which is:
        a. Slow and progressively painful disease
        b. Highly communicable and contagious
        c. Non-communicable and slowly contagious

574.   Choose the best answer that pertains to common causes of fainting:
        a. Emotional shock and overeating
        b. Emotional shock, overeating and sight of blood
        c. Emotional shock, sight of blood and too hot bath

575.   To render fist aid to a person who has fainted, you should:
        a. Elevate the legs or lays the person flat on the back with head lower than the rest of body
        b. Sit the person up in a chair and bend body forward and allow head to fall below the knees
        c. All of the above (A & B)

576.   The causes of panting are:
        a. The sight of blood, emotional shock and extreme pain
        b. Fainting and panting
        c. Head pain

577.   Favus is a:
     a. Fungus infection of the mouth
     b. Fungus infection of the stomach, usually the gall bladder
     c. Fungus infection of the skin, usually the scalp

578.   Felon is a bad and usually painful abscess found:
     a. At the opening of the eardrum
     b. At the tip of a finger
     c. On the breast

579.   To determine severity of someone's fever you need to know:
     a. How long has the fever been present, how high it has been and much it fluctuated
     b. If the person with the fever temperatures is moderating between low and high
     c. If the fever been present for more than three hours

580.   Fever blister is a:
     a. A rapid and contagious disease that need quick medical attention
     b. A contagious disease that needs a medical doctor
     c. A mild virus infection requiring no treatment

581.   Fibroid is a:
     a. Harmless tumor or new growth inside the uterus
     b. New growth of both white blood cells and red blood cells
     c. None of the above

582.   Fibula is one of the:
     a. Two bones of the upper leg
     b. Two bones of the lower leg
     c. Circular bones in the lower back

583.   Fish-skin disease known as ichthyosis is a:
     a. Skin blemish
     b. Skin rash
     c. Skin disorder

584.   Flatulence is the accumulation of:
 a. Bowel movement
 b. Gas or air on the stomach or in the bowels
 c. Atherosclerosis

585.   Flush is a:
 a. Reddening of skin on face and neck
 b. Puffiness under the eyelids
 c. The swelling under the chin

586   Fontanel is the:
 a. Hard spots on the human skull
 b. Joints that connect the skull to the body
 c. Soft spots on a baby's skull

587.   The usual symptoms of food poisoning are:
 a. Severe diarrhea and itchiness
 b. Severe vomiting, diarrhea and abdominal pain
 c. Severe itchiness and minor vomiting

588.   Herpes can be:
 a. Delicate, obsolete or contagious
 b. Highly delicate, contagious or non contagious
 c. Highly contagious, contagious or inactive

589.   Freckles are:
 a. Small yellow and brown pigmented spots on the skin
 b. Large yellow and brown-pigmented spots on people with lighter skin
 c. Small yellow spots that becomes noticeable with sun exposures

590.   People who appear to be subject to freckles are those with:
 a. Whiter skins, and often those with blonde hair
 b. Delicate skins, and often those with red hair
 c. Only visible to people who are teenagers or older

591.   Frog breathing is taught to patients with:
 a. Respiratory difficulty
 b. Urinary difficulty
 c. Overweight and exercising

592.   Frostbite results from:
    a. Exposure to cold and heat
    b. Exposure to severe cold
    c. Exposure to excessive heat

593.   Furuncle is a:
    a. Small boil
    b. Chemical burn
    c. Fungus

594.   Gangrene occurs when the circulation of blood to a part of the body is hampered due to damage damaged tissue so that:
    a. The tissue can no longer get nourishment
    b. The tissue cannot dispose of waste products
    c. All of the above (A & B)

595.   Dry gangrene occurs most commonly in:
    a. Older people and diabetics
    b. Younger children with bleeding
    c. Animals only

596.   Dry gangrene mostly affects older and diabetes people in what area of the body?
    a. The mouth
    b. Feet and toes
    c. Under the armpits

597.   In moist gangrene, the affected part is:
    a. Swollen, blistered, green or black in some areas
    b. Wanton, blue, red or black in all areas
    c. Blistered, green, yellow, red or black in all areas

598.   Gas on the stomach or in the bowels is called:
    a. Asphyxia
    b. Gastroenteritis
    c. Flatulence

599.   Another name for gastralgia is:
    a. Bellyache or stomach trouble
    b. Gas poisoning or asphyxia
    c. None of the above

600.   Hypoxia is:
    a. A deficiency of red blood cells in the body
    b. A deficiency of oxygen in the blood
    c. All of the above A & B

601.   Gastritis is:
    a. Inflammation of the bones
    b. Inflammation of the stomach
    c. Inflammation of the bile and uterus

602.   Geriatrics is a branch of medicine that specializes in:
    a. Disease and disabilities of young children
    b. Disease in animals
    c. Disease, disorder and disabilities of older people

603.   Gingivitis is:
    a. Inflammation of the bowel
    b. Inflammation of the gums
    c. Inflammation of the digestive organs

604.   Glucose is the form in which sugar usually appear in:
    a. The blood stream (blood sugar)
    b. Certain fruits (fruit sugar
    c. All of the above (A & B)

605.   Gonorrhea is a:
    a. Sexually transmitted disease
    b. Food poisoning
    c. Related to the gluteus muscles

606.   A goiter is:
    a. Animal starch stored in the liver
    b. An enlargement of the thyroid gland in the neck
    c. A kind of protein found on green leafy vegetables

607.   Green sickness is a nutritional anemia found in:
        a. Newborn babies
        b. Young teen-age boys
        c. Young teen-age girls

608.   Growing pains in children who complain of legs and back pains are:
        a. Rheumatic fever
        b. Flat feet and rapture spine
        c. None of the above

609.   Gynecomastia is:
        a. The enlargement of breasts in the male
        b. The enlargement of breasts in the female
        c. The enlargement of breasts in pregnant women

610.   Bloom syndrome is a condition in which children are:
        a. Prone to tumor of the brain and skull
        b. Small, grow poorly, and have frequent infections
        c. Usually overgrown due to hormone injections taken at a young age

611.   Another name for halitosis is:
        a. Hangover
        b. Foot trouble
        c. Bad breath

612.   The most common cause or halitosis is:
        a. Hallucination
        b. Infected teeth or gums
        c. None of the above

613.   Hallucination is a mental mirage of:
        a. Hearing, seeing or feeling things that are present
        b. Hearing, seeing or feeling things that are not really there
        c. Dreaming about things that are not really there in your sleep

614.   The heart is a hollow muscles that:
        a. Pumps blood through the blood vessels in all parts of the body
        b. Pumps sections of the heart and blood streams
        c. Pumps blood through sections of the arteries

615.   A heart healthy diet is:
    a. Low on saturated fat but rich in fruits, vegetables and whole grains
    b. High in saturated fat and trans fat but low in fruits, vegetables and whole grains
    c. High in proteins and carbohydrates, fructose, vegetables and enriched flour

616.   A damaged cardiovascular system is usually concentrated on:
    a. Lack of exercise and low cholesterol levels
    b. High in saturated fats and high blood pressure
    c. High blood pressure and high cholesterol levels

617.   Heat stroke is the result from:
    a. Exposure to excessive heat, indoor or outdoor
    b. Exposure to excessive outdoor heat
    c. Exposure to excessive sunlight

618.   Small hemorrhages are called:
    a. Petechial
    b. Blood secretion
    c. Hemophilia

619.   Hemophilia is known as:
    a. An obese disease
    b. A bleeder's disease
    c. A bleeder's healthiness

620.   Hermaphrodite is a person who is:
    a. Having only one testicle
    b. Half man and half woman where the sex organs are both male and female
    c. An animal that lives in the desert and are like scavengers

621.   Cerebral palsy is usually caused by:
    a. Too much stress on the pregnant mother
    b. Blood deficiency found in newborn babies
    c. Lack of oxygen to the brain

622.   Common occurrence in spina bifida:
    a. Spine and kidney problems
    b. Low blood pressure and kidney problems
    c. Bowel and bladder problems

623.   High blood pressure is a consistent elevation of:
    a. Eating low fiber diets and high carbohydrates into the blood vessels
    b. Blood pulsating against the walls of the arteries and other blood vessels
    c. Chemical imbalance that is pressed against the arteries of the blood vessels

624.   High blood pressure brings about other cardiovascular disorders such as:
    a. Heart disease, stroke and shortness of breath
    b. Stroke, heart disease, hardening of the joints and cardiovascular disorder
    c. Stroke, heart disease, kidney trouble and hardening of the arteries

625.   High blood pressure affects in which order:
    a. Blood vessels, kidney and heart
    b. Heart and blood vessels and then indirectly other organs
    c. Blood vessels, heart, kidney and other organs

626.   Hypoglycemia is:
    a. Having too little sugar in the blood
    b. Having too little red blood cells
    c. Having too much sugar in the blood streams

627.   Hysterectomy is:
    a. Surgical removal of the uterus
    b. Surgical removal of the vagina
    c. Surgical removal of the abdomen

628.   Your gums are swollen, redden and bleeding, it is a sign of:
    a. Gum pigmentation
    b. Gingivitis
    c. Inflammation from wearing braces and retaines

629.   When someone has an idiopathic disease, it means that:
    a. The doctor does not know what is causing it
    b. The doctor associates the disease with other causes
    c. The doctor recommends an allergy testing

630.   Ileus is:
    a. Brain obstruction
    b. Mouth obstruction
    c. Bowel obstruction

631.   Impetigo is a:
    a. Brain malfunction
    b. Ear infection
    c. Skin disorder

632.   Incontinence is the:
    a. Inability to hold back tears
    b. Inability to hold back urine or bowel movement
    c. Inability to hold back urine due to stomach cramps

633.   Infantie is referred to a:
    a. Child born with skin disease
    b. Child born with infectious eyes
    c. Childish; underdeveloped baby

634.   Influenza is a:
    a. Virus disease that may attack the respiratory, nervous or gastroin-
       testinal system
    b. Virus disease that usually attack the respiratory and nervous systems
    c. Fatal respiratory and virus disease that is very inflammatory

635.   The symptoms of influenza usually comes on:
    a. Slowly, anywhere from a period of 72 to 160 hours
    b. Gradually, after an incubation period of three to 12 hours
    c. Suddenly, after an incubation period of 12 to 72 hours

636.   The correct I.Q. measurement is:
a. 50 to 70 is dull, 70 to 90 is normal and over 125 is genius
b. 50 to 70 is mental deficiency, 70 to 90 is superior and above 140 is genius
c. 90 to 110 is normal, 110 to 125 is superior and above 140 is genius

637.   Intussusception is a peculiar form of:
a. Bowel obstruction, most common in infants
b. Bowel obstruction, most common in older people
c. Mild form of bowel obstruction

638.   Dyslexia is a specific learning disability that is:
a. Stubborn in nature
b. Neurological in origin
c. Learned by practicing

639.   Ketogenic is a diet rich in:
a. Fats, low in carbohydrates, intended to produce ketone in the blood and urine
b. Proteins, low in carbohydrates, intended to produce ketone in the blood and urine
c. Carbohydrates and fats, low in protein, intended to produce ketone in the blood and urine

640.   Kidney stones, a common form of kidney trouble:
a. Often is painful and an urgent operation must be carried out
b. Often obstruct the passing of urine by infecting the bladder
c. Often induce bladder trouble and infections in the urinary system

641.   The most common signs of kidney trouble is:
a. Painful experienced when urinating
b. Difficulties in urination and abnormalities of urine
c. Abnormalities of urine in the bladder

642.   Laryngitis is:
a. The popular name for nitrous oxide
b. The medical specialty that deals with disease and disorders of the throat
c. Inflammation of the larynx, denotes by hoarseness and dryness of the throat

643.   Leptospirosis is a disease caused by a spirochete, and is carried by:
    a. Rats, dogs, cows and other animals
    b. A reduction in the red blood cells
    c. Sleeping with someone who has the leptospirosis disease

644.   If someone is lethargic it usually means that the person:
    a. Suffers a serious breakdown in blood count
    b. Has a tired feeling
    c. Hard of hearing in one ear

645.   Mental retardation can occur:
    a. Before birth
    b. Before or after birth
    c. Before, during or after birth

646.   Leukemia is sometimes called:
    a. Caner of the mouth
    b. Cancer of the blood
    c. Cancer of the bowel

647.   Leukemia is a:
    a. Fatal disease
    b. Dietary disease
    c. Harmless disease

648.   Leukemia disease may:
    a. Progress slowly or rapidly
    b. Chronic or acute
    c. All of the above (A & B)

649.   Someone who has leukopenia it means the person has:
    a. An increase in the number of circulating red blood cells
    b. A decrease in the number of circulating white blood cells
    c. An increase in the number of circulating white blood cells

650.   Lipoma is a:
    a. A male sex organ, usually in overweight men
    b. Tumor in the brain
    c. Fatty tumor, usually painless and harmless

651.   The lymphoid organs are divided into the primary and secondary groups. The primary lymphoid organs are:
a. The bone marrow and thymus gland
b. The lungs and thymus gland
c. The lymph modes and lymph gland

652.   A mantoux test is a sample and common test used in:
a. Jaundice case finding
b. Tuberculosis case-finding
c. Cancerous growth

653.   Mastalgia is referred to as:
a. Pain in the breasts
b. Pain in the buttocks
c. Pain in the uterus

654.   Mastication is the:
a. Act of swelling of the joints
b. Act of belching
c. Act of chewing food

655.   Mastitis is referred to as:
a. Inflammation of the groin
b. Inflammation of the bowel
c. Inflammation of the breasts

656.   The measles disease is most contagious in the:
a. Early stages from about 4 days before and up 5 days after the appearance of the rash
b. Late stages from about 10 days before until 30 days after the appearance of the rash
c. Early stages from about one day before until 20 days after the appearance of the rash

657.   Meningitis is inflammation of the meninges that:
a. Is associated to food poisoning
b. Envelop the pulmonary arteries and liver
c. Envelop the brain and spinal cord

658.   Meningococcal Meningitis is an acute infectious disease:
   a. Usually of sudden onset and in epidemic circumstances
   b. Usually of rare and gradual onset and in epidemic circumstances
   c. Usually slow and gradual onset and infectious circumstances

659.   Menopause relates to the:
   a. Time when a mother gives birth
   b. Time when normal menstruation starts
   c. Time when normal menstruation ceases

660.   The average age of menopause onset is:
   a. Age 39 to 44
   b. Age 45 to 49
   c. Age 50 to 55

661.   Menopause transition period may last:
   a. 2 or 3 years
   b. 4 or 5 years
   c. 6 or 7 years

662.   Symptoms of menopause may cause:
   a. Hot flashes, heart pain and loss of appetite
   b. Hot flashes, loss of mobility and appetite
   c. Hot flashes, fatigue and depression

663.   Menorrhagia is:
   a. Profuse menstrual bleeding
   b. Scanty menstrual bleeding
   c. Irregular menstrual bleeding

664.   Menstruation continues unless interrupted by:
   a. Pregnancy, miscarriage, early thirties to late thirties
   b. Pregnancy or disease or until menopause
   c. Pregnancy or late thirties to early forties when menopause sets in

665.   Metrorrhagia is:
   a. Normal menstrual bleeding
   b. Abnormal uterine bleeding not associated with menstruation
   c. The spread of menstrual disease

666. Migraine, is generally confined to:
    a. All over the head
    b. The abdomen
    c. One side of the head

667. The minerals most likely to be deficient in diets are:
    a. Calcium, iron and magnesium
    b. Calcium, potassium, and sulfur
    c. Calcium, iron and iodine

668. Another name for miscarriage is:
    a. Spontaneous abortion
    b. Childbirth
    c. Misinterpretation of pregnancy

669. Moles are:
    a. Skin abnormalities
    b. Bowel abnormalities
    c. Pregnancy abnormalities

670. An enlarging mole may be a forerunner of:
    a. Stomach enlargement and should get prompt attention
    b. Skin cancer and should always get prompt attention
    c. Minor bowel enlargement and should get prompt attention

671. A 'Monster' is:
    a. An adult with horns growing out of his or head
    b. An animal that is so dangerous that it has to be caved up
    c. A badly deformed fetus, if born, usually lack vital parts such as heart or head

672. Mortality is:
    a. The ratio number of deaths to the total population
    b. The ratio number of casualties to the total population
    c. The ratio number of sick people to the total population

673.   Motion sickness is associated with:
a. Dizziness, vomiting, hunger and long rides
b. Dizziness, headache, nausea and vomiting
c. Dizziness, nausea, vomiting and sleepiness

674.   Symptoms accompanying an allergic reaction can be:
a. Aching stomach, rash, itching, hives and throat virus
b. Bowel disease in the stomach caused by lack of regular bowel movement
c. Itching, rash, nasal congestion, weeping eyes or coughing

675.   The Multiple sclerosis (MS) virus is acquired:
a. Late in life and causes a rapid progressive viral infection in a short time
b. Late in life and causes a slow, progressive immobility over time
c. Early in life and causes a slow, progressive viral infection over time

676.   The signs and symptoms of Multiple sclerosis (MS) are:
a. Muscle weakness, bowel movement, pain in the joints
b. Muscle weakness, blurred vision, confusion and anxiety
c. Muscle weakness, stiffness of the joints and joint inflammation

677.   Multiple sclerosis is a:
a. Chronic, relapsing neurological, crippling disease of the central nervous system
b. Sometimes chronic, but not crippling disease of the vascular system
c. Nasal congestion that is imminent during the cold months

678.   The most common symptom of MS is:
a. Relapsing
b. Sleeping
c. Fatigue

679.   Mumps is an:
a. Incision found on the thyroid
b. Acute contagious disease
c. Arch found on baby's feet

680. The identified characteristic of Mumps are:
   a. Inflammation, swelling, and tenderness of the parotid glands
   b. The swelling of the arch on the baby's feet
   c. Swelling around the groin, marked by tenderness and unable to urinate

681. Mumps is essentially a:
   a. Young infant disease, occurring between the ages of three months to 23 months
   b. Childhood disease, occurring between the ages of 5 to 15
   c. Young adult disease, occurring between the ages of 16 to 25

682. Mumps incubation period ranges from:
   a. 5 days to a week
   b. 12 to 26 days
   c. 30 to 40 days

683. When a muscle's nerve supply is interrupted, the muscle becomes:
   a. Paralyzed
   b. Frail during the cooler months
   c. Soft and little strength in the arm

684. Constant practice and graded exercise are essential to:
   a. Maintaining of muscular skills and development
   b. Maintaining of muscular biceps and skills
   c. Producing energy toward muscular movements

685. Muscular dystrophy is a:
   a. Progressive symptom that keeps the voluntary muscles firm
   b. Progressive symptom that destroys the muscular built and tissues in the body
   c. Progressive disease that destroys the striped or striated voluntary muscles

686. For anyone to stay well, the mind influences:
   a. The brain
   b. The immune system
   c. The nervous system

687.   Muscular dystrophy affects more … between … and … years:
 a. Boys … 2 and 5
 b. Girls … 2 and 5
 c. Both boys and girls … 2 and 5

688.   To experience myasthenia it means that the person is experiencing:
 a. Muscular weakness
 b. Eye trouble, a sing of failing vision
 c. Piles or hemorrhoids in the varicose veins

689.   Myelitis relates to:
 a. Inflammation of the muscles
 b. Inflammation of the spinal cord
 c. Inflammation of the heart muscles

690.   Myeloma is any:
 a. Abnormal growth of white blood cells
 b. Abnormal growth of cells found in the blood vessels
 c. Abnormal growth of cells found in the bone marrow

691.   Amyotrophic lateral sclerosis (ALS) is often referred to as:
 a. "Gingivitis disease"
 b. "Scarlet fever disese"
 c. "Lou Gehrig's disease"

692.   The four classes of narcotics are:
 a. Opium, cocaine, barbiturates and marijuana
 b. Potassium, opium, nasopharynx and cocaine
 c. None of the above

693.   Foods with flavanoids that have natural antioxidants that contain anti-inflammatory substances are:
 a. Bananas, morphine, natural orange juice, water and brown bread
 b. Nuts, grapes, cranberries, onions, tomatoes, red wine and tea
 c. Opium, white wine, nuts, orange juice, apricot and basil leaves

694.   The most dangerous drugs of morphine, codeine, papaverine and heroin is:
a. Papaverine
b. Morphine
c. Heroin

695.   Neisserian is a:
a. Stomach flu
b. Venereal disease
c. Parts of the nervous system

696.   A surgical removal of a kidney is called:
a. Hysterectomy
b. Nephrectomy
c. Sterilization

697.   Nephritis is the sign of:
a. Drug overdose
b. Damaged nerve cells
c. Inflammation in the kidneys

698.   The human nervous system has three main divisions. They are:
a. Central, autonomic and peripheral nervous systems
b. Central, outer and inner nervous systems
c. Top, middle and lower nervous systems

699.   The central nervous system consists of the:
a. Brain, spinal cord and their interconnections
b. Head, brain and interconnections
c. Brain, cell body and peripheral nervous tissues

700.   The brain is the largest and most specialized mass of:
a. Brain compartment in the human body
b. Nerve cells in the human body
c. Inner nervous system in the human body

701.   Neuralgia is a pain in a nerve. Select the answer that correctly describes neuralgia:
a. Ulcer
b. Arthritics pain
c. A toothache

702.   A surgical specialist trained to operate on the nervous system and the brain is called:
a. Neurosurgeon
b. Neuropsychiatrist
c. Neurologist

703.   If someone has a neutropenia it means that person has:
a. Hallucination
b. Brain tumor
c. White blood cell disease

704.   Nicotine is the principal active alkaloid in:
a. Vitamin B complex
b. Tobacco
c. Acid

705.   If a person has bipolar disorder it means that:
a. The person has severe mood swings
b. The person has a degree of polio
c. The person has increased blood supply going to the brain

706.   The life-essential process of assimilating food or nutriment is:
a. Nutrition
b. Diet
c. Weight watching

707.   Obesity causes extra burden on your:
a. Stomach and legs
b. Heart and circulation system
c. Feet and digestive systems

708.   On an average, obese people die:
    a. Earlier than the normal underweight person
    b. Later than the normal and underweight person
    c. Die the same time as the normal and underweight person

709.   The medical specialty of managing the conditions related to childbirth
    is called:
    a. An occupational therapist
    b. An obstetrics
    c. An ophthalmologist or oculist

710.   When someone is oliguria it means that the person:
    a. Cannot sleep with taking sleeping pills
    b. Needs high dosage of lanolin ointment
    c. Scanty urine

711.   Osteoporosis is having:
    a. Too much weight on the lower body
    b. Porous bone
    c. Medical eye condition

712.   Ovulation occurs at about:
    a. Beginning point of the menstrual cycle
    b. Midpoint of the menstrual cycle
    c. End point o f the menstrual cycle

713.   The warning siren that some part of the body is under stress or attack is:
    a. Diarrhea
    b. Humor
    c. Pain

714.   Papanicolaou is another name for:
    a. Pap smear, to detect diseases of the uterine cervix
    b. Papaverine, a narcotic drugs
    c. Pancreas, a long organ or gland

715   Paralysis is the:
    a. Loss of muscle function, usually to a damaged nerve
    b. Milder form of typhoid fever
    c. Walls of any body cavity, usually the skull

716.   Parkinson's disease is a degenerative disease in which something goes wrong with the:
    a. Eye ganglia
    b. Parotid glands
    c. Nerve ganglia

717.   Pelvic diseases usually refer to some:
    a. Male diseases
    b. Female diseases
    c. Animal diseases

718.   Penis is the:
    a. Female organ of copulation and urinary system
    b. Male organ of copulation and urination
    c. Name given to the private part of the human body

719.   A normal means of regulation of the body temperature is by:
    a. Perspiration or drinking
    b. Sweating or steam shower
    c. Perspiration or sweating

720.   Phobia is someone who experience:
    a. An abnormal fear
    b. Fatigue
    c. Procaine

721.   The best sources of protein in the human diet are:
    a. Vegetables, eggs, juice and milk products such as cheese
    b. Poultry, beans, potatoes, white bread, rice and cheese
    c. Meat, eggs, nuts, milk and milk products such as cheese

722. Inflammation of the kidney—usually its inner core or pelvis is called a:
   a. Surrogate
   b. Pyelitis
   c. Kidney pain

723. A paralysis where all four extremities; both hands and legs are missing:
   a. Handicapped
   b. Spinal cord injury
   c. Quadriplegia

724. A viral disease, usually fatal, transmitted from animals is known as:
   a. Flu
   b. Rabies
   c. Dengue fever

725. Inflammation at the root of the nerve is referred to:
   a. Radiculitis
   b. Ramus
   c. None of the above

726. To get sicker after being better is called a:
   a. Relapse
   b. Lethargic
   c. Remission

727. The disappearance of signs and symptoms of diseases without the eradication of the primary cause of the disease is called a:
   a. Relapse
   b. Remission
   c. Renal

728. Which best describes rheumatism:
   a. Aches and pains in the muscles, bones and joints
   b. Aches and pains in the stomach, anus and joints
   c. Pains in the head, throat, stomach, bones and muscles

729.   Inflammation, usually with some swelling, of the lining of the nose is known as:
a. Nose bleed
b. Rhinitis
c. Sinus trouble

730.   A common garden plant, sometimes used as an herb remedy and serves as a mild laxative:
a. Ivy
b. Texan herb
c. Rhubarb

731.   Bacteria which is sometimes responsible for food poisoning:
a. Salmonella
b. Potassium nitrate
c. Pernio

732.   Which emotions do not serve any purpose in your life?
a. Anger, guilt, fear, and worry
b. Skin blemish, tone, and hope
c. Prayer, hope and aspiration

733.   Schizophrenia is a:
a. Skin disease
b. Mental illness
c. Mental symptom

734.   In schizophrenia the victim suffer from:
a. Delusions
b. Hallucinations
c. Delusions and hallucinations

735.   Complete the following sentence. Delusions are.... Hallucinations are …
a. True and predetermined ideas. Hallucinations are imaginary voices and real visions
b. Delusion is false and voluntary ideas. Hallucinations are real and visions are imaginary
c. Delusions are false and fixed ideas. Hallucinations are imaginary voices and visions

736.   Scurvy is a:
a. Protein deficiency disease, lacking vitamin A
b. Vitamin deficiency disease, lacking vitamin C
c. Blood deficiency disease, lacking vitamin C

737.   An infantile paralysis, and infectious disease that sometimes kills and
sometimes cripples is called:
a. Polio
b. Piles
c. Ulcer

738   In the 4th month of pregnancy, the embryo is called a:
a. Miscarriage
b. Termination
c. Fetus

739.   The 5th month of pregnancy, real hair appears on the:
a. Head of the fetus
b. Eyebrow of the fetus
c. Body of the fetus

740.   The 6th month of pregnancy, the fetus':
a. Brain is recording things in the womb
b. Eyes open
c. Eat

741.   A common name for placenta is:
a. Cicatrix
b. Codeine
c. Afterbirth

742.   The first Polio vaccine is given at:
a. Three to six months
b. Six to twelve months
c. Twelve to twenty-four months

743   During pregnancy one experiences:
    a. Breast tenderness, fatigue and urinary urgency
    b. Urinary urgency, impotency and bleeding
    c. Food intake, breast tenderness and diabetes

744.   During pregnancy calories intake should:
    a. Increase to about 50 calories per day
    b. Increase to about 300 calories per day
    c. Increase to about 1,200 calories per day

745.   To meet the nutritional demands of pregnancy, a diet consisting of:
    a. 900 calories per day depending on age is required
    b. 1500 calories per day depending on age is required
    c. 2500 calories per day depending on age is required

746.   Peripheral arterial disease (PAD) occurs most often in the:
    a. Head
    b. Stomach
    c. Legs

747.   The blood test used for early detection of prostate cancer in men is called:
    a. Prostate specific antigen (PSA)
    b. Magnetic Resonance Imaging
    c. Gastrointestinal Imaging

748.   The treatment used to clean your blood when your kidneys fail is:
    a. Biologist
    b. Dialysis
    c. Hormones replacement

749.   Bone Mineral Density testing is used in early detection of:
    a. Osteoporosis
    b. Multiple Sclerosis
    c. Angina

750.   There are no known medical detection or cure for:
    a. Ventriculogram
    b. Diabetes
    c. Autism

751.   The seafood with the highest omega-3 fatty acids, which can decrease triglycerides and thins the blood naturally is:
    a. Salmon, chicken and beans
    b. Salmon, cod and bass fish
    c. Chicken, beans and ginger

752.   High levels of glucose may indicate:
    a. Diabetes mellitus
    b. Multiple sclerosis
    c. Osteoporosis

753.   Failure to change lifestyle habits contribute to:
    a. Chronic illness, such as glaucoma, heartburns, kidney infection and warts
    b. Forgetfulness, pain in your legs, obesity, ulitis disease and osmotic pressure
    c. Chronic illness, especially obesity, cancer, heart disease and diabetes

754.   Obesity may soon cause as much preventable disease and death as:
    a. Motor vehicle accidents
    b. Cigarette smoking
    c. Scarlet fever

755.   Biopsies are used to determine whether abnormal tissue is:
    a. Malignant (cancerous) or benign (non-cancerous)
    b. Reticulitis (inflammation) or radium (rare)
    c. Acute (severe) or extreme or insignificant

756.   Biopsies are also used to determine the cause of a problem such as:
    a. Arthritis or pulled ligaments
    b. Bacterial or viral infection or inflammation
    c. Miscarriage or spontaneous abortion

757.   Endoscopy is a procedure that permits a doctor to examine the:
    a. Muscle tract
    b. Nervous system tract
    c. Gastrointestinal tract

758.   To investigate the large intestine (a colonoscopy) or the esophagus, stomach and upper intestine the patient must have this procedure:
a. An endoscopy
b. Mammogram
c. PET scan

759.   Symptoms of an under-active thyroid includes:
a. Tiredness, constipation and sensitivity to the cold
b. Belly aches, diarrhea and sensitivity to the heat
c. Tiredness, diarrhea and enhanced appetite

760.   An x-ray that is used to detect the presence of tumors or cysts in the breast tissue is called
a. A Biopsy
b. A Mammogram
c. An EEG or Electroencephalogram

761.   Match the correct answer:
a. Multiple sclerosis patients see a neurologist and diabetes see an endocrinologist
b. Multiple sclerosis patients see a dermatologist and diabetes see a gynecologist
c. Multiple sclerosis patients see a pharmacologist and diabetes see a neurologist

762.   The best way to managing diabetes or osteoporosis is:
a. Drink plenty of water, lactic acid and eat lots of carbohydrates
b. Sleeping for at least eight hours a day
c. Developing healthy habits like regular exercise

763.   Stage I hypertension or high blood pressure is:
a. 140/90 or higher
b. 120/80 or lower
c. 110/70 or higher

764.   Poor eating habits and excess weight can:
a. Give MS patients pressure ulcers
b. Aggravate MS symptoms
c. Let MS patients get much more tired

765.   Having MS is a strong risk factor for:
       a. Blood clotting
       b. Hemorrhoids (piles)
       c. Osteoporosis (bone loss)

766.   Pressure ulcers, also known as decubitus ulcers is caused by anyone who:
       a. Eats and then lay down shortly afterward
       b. Sits or lays most of the day
       c. Eats irregular (skips meals)

767.   The skin can be nourished by:
       a. Nourishing creams and lotions
       b. Contour cream and skin conditioner
       c. Vitamin A and Riboflavin

768.   Narcolepsy is:
       a. People who can't help falling asleep during the day
       b. People who can't help not waking up and eating during the night
       c. People who is overdosed on narcotic drugs

769.   Varicose veins occur because of:
       a. Uneven flow of the blood to the veins and valves congestion
       b. Weakening walls of the veins or valves and venous congestion
       c. Excessive weight on the feet, veins and valves congestion

770.   Better eating habits arc those found in children who eat:
       a. Foods low in saturated fat but high in cholesterol
       b. Foods high in saturated fat and high in cholesterol
       c. Foods low in saturated fat and low in cholesterol

771.   Inflammation of the tissue of the mouth, usually including the gums is called:
       a. Toothache
       b. Lymph Nodes
       c. Stomatitis

772.   Coronary artery disease is a condition in which the coronary arteries become:
a. Narrowed and rigid
b. Deep and firm
c. Lessened and strong

773.   The best normal blood pressure reading is:
a. 75/60
b. 100/70
c. 120/80

774.   … is a serious eye disease
a. Trachoma
b. Ulcer
c. Eye irritation

775.   Abnormalities of urination usually signal:
a. Pregnancy
b. Disease
c. Bedwetting

776.   Scanty urination may depict:
a. Serious bedwetting
b. Serious kidney trouble
c. Venereal disease

777.   Avocado, peach, baked potato with skin on and banana will:
a. Increase your appetite
b. Reduce blood pressure
c. Reduce weight gain

778.   Orange juice, spinach, and folic acid will:
a. Reduce cancer
b. Reduce high blood pressure
c. Reduce constipation

779. Cauliflower, broccoli and cabbage will help to:
    a. Prevent wrinkles
    b. Prevent aging
    c. Prevent cancer

780. Warning signs of cancer include:
    a. Nagging cough or hoarseness; unusual bleeding
    b. Indigestion or difficulty swallowing; lumps in the breast
    c. All of the above (A & B)

781. Cardiovascular disease, known as CVD is a collection of diseases and conditions of the heart and blood vessels including:
    a. Angina, atherosclerosis, hypertension and stroke
    b. Angina, hypertension, cauterization and stroke
    c. Urethral, heart failure, hypertension, osteoporosis

782. It is estimated that the common cold has:
    a. 50 or more different viruses
    b. 100 or more different viruses
    c. 200 or more different viruses

783. To lower cholesterol levels you must avoid foods with:
    a. High content of saturated fat, cholesterol and trans fatty acids
    b. Low content of saturated fat, cholesterol and trans fatty acids
    c. None of the above

784. Emergency preparedness for burn includes:
    a. Covering burns with ice
    b. Covering burns with cool cloth
    c. Covering burns with petroleum jelly

785. The percentage of illnesses caused by stress is:
    a. Twenty (20) percent
    b. Fifty (50) percent
    c. Eighty (80) percent

786.   The symptoms of low blood sugar (hypoglycemia) is:
    a. Sweating, blurred vision, dizziness and hunger
    b. Not feeling hungry, low heart rate and fatigue
    c. All of the above A & B

787.   The number one killer for newborn babies in America is:
    a. Spinal cord injury
    b. Caesarian birth
    c. Premature birth

788.   Women should visit their gynecologists to get a PAP smear test for cancer:
    a. Once a month
    b. Once a year
    c. Once every five years

789.   Good cholesterol (HDL) levels are…. and bad cholesterol (LDL) levels are:
    a. HDL are 40 mg/dl or less and LDL are 160 mg/dl or more
    b. HDL are 200 mg/dl or more and LDL 180 mg/dl or less
    c. None of the above

790.   Symptoms of Asthma attacks are:
    a. Wheezing, coughing, laughing and sneezing
    b. Wheezing, coughing, chest tightness and shortness of breath
    c. Wheezing, coughing, sneezing and fatty acids

791.   The following can trigger asthma attacks:
    a. Heartburns, pets, molds or pollen
    b. Pets, bottled water or high cholesterol level
    c. Pollens, pets, sweaty glands or HIV/AIDS virus

792.   To protect yourself from catching the flu virus from someone, you should:
    a. Wash hands, have a hot cup of soup at least once a week
    b. Keep your distance, hug no one and drink a glass of wine a day
    c. Keep your distance, wash hands and maintain healthy lifestyle

793.   By laughing the body releases:
       a. Enzymes
       b. Veratrum
       c. Endorphins

794.   The acronym AIDS stands for:
       a. Acquired Immunity Deficiency Symptoms
       b. Acquired Immune Deficiency Syndrome
       c. Ascribed Immunodeficiency Syndrome

795.   ALS is a progressive neurodengenerative disease that attacks the:
       a. Nerve cells in the brain and spinal cord
       b. The spinal cord to the muscles throughout the body
       c. All of the above (A & B)

796.   Cancer sites are:
       a. Skin, uterus, breast, rectum, lung, stomach, larynx and mouth
       b. Head, skin, breast, jaw, rectum, lung, stomach, comedo and mouth
       c. Lung, skin, stomach, larynx, eye, radium, hermaphrodite and mouth

797.   Blood pressure risk factors you can change are:
       a. Multiple sclerosis, memory loss, obesity, wrinkles and old age
       b. Obesity, lack of exercise, stress, high salt intake and smoking
       c. Cancer, multiple sclerosis, depression, wrinkles and smoking

798.   Stroke warning signs are:
       a. Trouble sleeping, eating, lack of appetite and weakness in the joints
       b. Difficulty exercising, pain in the chest and lack of sleep
       c. Sudden numbness or weakness, trouble speaking and loss of balance

799.   Blood is carried from the heart to all parts of the body in vessels through:
       a. Arteries
       b. Batteries
       c. Culinary

800.   The fastest growing serious developmental disability in the U.S. in 2006
was:
a. Autism
b. Biopsy
c. Colon cancer

SECTION VI

This is section six, and it provides the Answer Charts, where all the answers for each question is located, from one through to eight hundred. Also included in this section are: The score cards, rating sheets, postscript, find a word puzzle, how to purchase a book without the board game and certificate.

ANSWER CHARTS

The answer charts have one hundred answers per chart, and are divided into three sections, as seen below. Answers 1 to 200 contain the beginners level; 201 to 400 intermediate level and 401 through to 800 for the advanced level. Players can use the charts to check their answers against the *Healthiology 101* quiz game book.

1. Beginner: 1–200

2. Intermediate: 201–400

3. Advance: 401–600 and 601–800

Chart One: 1–200
Beginners Answers

1	B	26	A	51	A	76	C	101	C	126	C	151	A	176	C
2	C	27	C	52	C	77	B	102	A	127	C	152	A	177	A
3	A	28	B	53	A	78	B	103	C	128	C	153	B	178	B
4	B	29	C	54	B	79	A	104	A	129	A	154	C	179	B
5	A	30	A	55	B	80	C	105	B	130	B	155	A	180	B
6	B	31	A	56	C	81	C	106	B	131	B	156	B	181	A
7	B	32	B	57	A	82	B	107	C	132	C	157	A	182	C
8	A	33	A	58	C	83	B	108	A	133	A	158	C	183	B
9	A	34	B	59	C	84	B	109	C	134	B	159	C	184	A
10	B	35	C	60	B	85	B	110	C	135	A	160	A	185	A
11	C	36	C	61	C	86	C	111	B	136	C	161	C	186	B
12	B	37	A	62	B	87	B	112	B	137	B	162	A	187	C
13	B	38	A	63	C	88	A	113	C	138	A	163	B	188	B
14	C	39	B	64	B	89	C	114	A	139	B	164	B	189	A
15	B	40	C	65	A	90	B	115	C	140	C	165	B	190	C
16	C	41	A	66	B	91	C	116	A	141	C	166	A	191	B
17	B	42	C	67	C	92	C	117	C	142	B	167	A	192	B
18	B	43	A	68	A	93	B	118	C	143	A	168	B	193	B
19	C	44	B	69	B	94	C	119	A	144	C	169	A	194	C
20	C	45	C	70	A	95	A	120	B	145	C	170	B	195	B
21	A	46	B	71	C	96	B	121	B	146	B	171	A	196	A
22	B	47	A	72	B	97	C	122	B	147	A	172	B	197	C
23	C	48	C	73	C	98	B	123	A	148	A	173	C	198	A
24	B	49	B	74	C	99	B	124	C	149	C	174	A	199	B
25	C	50	B	75	B	100	A	125	A	150	B	175	C	200	A

Chart Two: 201–400
Intermediate Answers

201	B	226	B	251	B	276	B	301	A	326	A	351	C	376	A
202	C	227	C	252	A	277	C	302	C	327	B	352	A	377	C
203	C	228	A	253	C	278	A	303	C	328	C	353	B	378	C
204	A	229	B	254	B	279	A	304	A	329	B	354	C	379	C
205	C	230	C	255	C	280	B	305	B	330	C	355	B	380	B
206	B	231	C	256	C	281	B	306	A	331	A	356	A	381	A
207	A	232	A	257	B	282	A	307	B	332	C	357	C	382	A
208	C	233	C	258	A	283	B	308	A	333	C	358	B	383	C
209	C	234	C	259	C	284	A	309	A	334	B	359	C	384	B
210	A	235	A	260	B	285	B	310	C	335	C	360	B	385	B
211	C	236	B	261	C	286	C	311	B	336	C	361	B	386	C
212	C	237	A	262	A	287	C	312	A	337	B	362	A	387	A
213	B	238	A	263	C	288	B	313	A	338	A	363	C	388	B
214	A	239	B	264	A	289	C	314	C	339	A	364	C	389	B
215	A	240	C	265	A	290	A	315	B	340	C	365	B	390	A
216	C	241	A	266	C	291	B	316	A	341	B	366	B	391	C
217	C	242	A	267	C	292	C	317	B	342	B	367	C	392	C
218	B	243	C	268	A	293	B	318	A	343	A	368	A	393	B
219	C	244	A	269	B	294	A	319	C	344	C	369	A	394	B
220	A	245	B	270	C	295	B	320	C	345	B	370	B	395	A
221	C	246	A	271	B	296	C	321	A	346	C	371	C	396	B
222	C	247	B	272	A	297	C	322	C	347	B	372	B	397	C
223	B	248	C	273	A	298	A	323	C	348	A	373	C	398	A
224	A	249	B	274	A	299	B	324	A	349	A	374	B	399	B
225	C	250	C	275	B	300	A	325	C	350	B	375	C	400	C

Chart Three: 401–600
Advanced Answers

401	B	426	C	451	C	476	A	501	C	526	B	551	B	576	A
402	A	427	B	452	A	477	C	502	B	527	C	552	B	577	C
403	A	428	C	453	B	478	B	503	C	528	A	553	A	578	B
404	C	429	A	454	C	479	C	504	C	429	C	554	B	579	A
405	C	430	A	455	B	480	A	505	A	530	B	555	B	580	C
406	A	431	B	456	A	481	C	506	C	531	B	556	A	581	A
407	C	432	C	457	B	482	C	507	A	532	B	557	C	582	B
408	A	433	A	458	C	483	A	508	C	533	C	558	C	583	C
409	C	434	C	459	C	484	B	509	A	534	B	559	B	584	B
410	A	435	C	460	B	485	C	510	B	535	A	560	C	585	A
411	A	436	A	461	A	486	B	511	C	536	A	561	A	586	C
412	C	437	B	462	C	487	A	512	B	537	C	562	B	587	B
413	C	438	C	463	A	488	B	513	A	538	A	563	C	588	C
414	C	439	B	464	B	489	C	514	C	539	C	564	B	589	A
415	A	440	C	465	C	490	B	515	B	540	B	565	C	590	B
416	B	441	B	466	B	491	A	516	A	541	C	566	A	591	A
417	B	442	C	467	A	492	A	517	B	542	B	567	C	592	B
418	A	443	B	468	B	493	B	518	C	543	A	568	A	593	A
419	B	444	A	469	C	494	C	519	B	544	B	569	B	594	C
420	A	445	C	470	B	495	A	520	C	545	A	570	B	595	A
421	A	446	A	471	C	496	A	521	B	546	B	571	C	596	B
422	B	447	C	472	B	497	C	522	C	547	C	572	B	597	A
423	A	448	A	473	A	498	C	523	A	548	A	573	B	598	C
424	C	449	B	474	B	499	C	524	C	549	B	574	C	599	A
425	B	450	C	475	C	500	B	525	C	550	C	575	C	600	B

Chart Four: 601–800
Advanced Answers

601	B	626	A	651	A	676	B	701	C	726	A	751	B	776	B
602	C	627	A	652	B	677	A	702	A	727	B	752	A	777	B
603	B	628	B	653	A	678	C	703	C	728	A	753	C	778	A
604	C	629	A	654	C	679	B	704	B	729	B	754	B	779	C
605	A	630	C	655	C	680	A	705	A	730	C	755	A	780	C
606	B	631	C	656	A	681	B	706	A	731	A	756	B	781	A
607	C	632	B	657	C	682	B	707	B	732	A	757	C	782	C
608	A	633	C	658	A	683	A	708	A	733	B	758	A	783	A
609	A	634	A	659	C	684	A	709	B	734	C	759	A	784	B
610	B	635	C	660	B	685	C	710	C	735	C	760	B	785	C
611	C	636	C	661	A	686	B	711	B	736	B	761	A	786	A
612	B	637	A	662	C	687	A	712	B	737	A	762	C	787	C
613	B	638	B	663	A	688	A	713	C	738	C	763	A	788	B
614	A	639	A	664	B	689	B	714	A	739	A	764	B	789	A
615	A	640	C	665	B	690	C	715	A	740	B	765	C	790	B
616	C	641	B	666	C	691	C	716	C	741	C	766	B	791	A
617	A	642	C	667	C	692	A	717	B	742	B	767	C	792	C
618	A	643	A	668	A	693	B	718	B	743	A	768	A	793	C
619	B	644	B	669	A	694	C	719	C	744	B	769	B	794	B
620	B	645	C	670	B	695	B	720	A	745	C	770	C	795	C
621	C	646	B	671	C	696	B	721	C	746	C	771	C	796	A
622	C	647	A	672	A	697	C	722	B	747	A	772	A	797	B
623	B	648	C	673	B	698	A	723	C	748	B	773	C	798	C
624	C	649	B	674	C	699	A	724	B	749	A	774	A	799	A
625	B	650	C	675	C	700	B	725	A	750	C	775	B	800	A

HEALTHIOLOGY PLAYERS ACCOUNT SCORE CARD

Player:_____   Player: _____

Game #	Question #	Answer Here	Health Credit	Health Debit	Health Balance		Game #	Question #	Answer Here	Health Credit	Health Debit	Health Balance
1							1					
2							2					
3							3					
4							4					
5							5					
6							6					
7							7					
8							8					
9							9					
10							10					
11							11					
12							12					
13							13					
14							14					
15							15					
16							16					
17							17					
18							18					
19							19					
20							20					
21							21					
22							22					
23							23					
24							24					
25							25					
26							26					
27							27					
28							28					
28							29					
30							30					

Copy form for additional recording

HEALTHIOLOGY PLAYERS ACCOUNT
SCORE CARD

Player: _____   Player: _____

Game #	Question #	Answer Here	Health Credit	Health Debit	Health Balance		Game #	Question #	Answer Here	Health Credit	Health Debit	Health Balance
1							1					
2							2					
3							3					
4							4					
5							5					
6							6					
7							7					
8							8					
9							9					
10							10					
11							11					
12							12					
13							13					
14							14					
15							15					
16							16					
17							17					
18							18					
19							19					
20							20					
21							21					
22							22					
23							23					
24							24					
25							25					
26							26					
27							27					
28							28					
28							29					
30							30					

Copy form for additional recording

HEALTHIOLOGY PLAYERS ACCOUNT SCORE CARD

Player: _____   Player: _____

Game #	Question #	Answer Here	Health Credit	Health Debit	Health Balance		Game #	Question #	Answer Here	Health Credit	Health Debit	Health Balance
1							1					
2							2					
3							3					
4							4					
5							5					
6							6					
7							7					
8							8					
9							9					
10							10					
11							11					
12							12					
13							13					
14							14					
15							15					
16							16					
17							17					
18							18					
19							19					
20							20					
21							21					
22							22					
23							23					
24							24					
25							25					
26							26					
27							27					
28							28					
28							29					
30							30					

Copy form for additional recording

HEALTHIOLOGY PLAYERS ACCOUNT SCORE CARD

Player: _____   Player: _____

Game #	Question #	Answer Here	Health Credit	Health Debit	Health Balance		Game #	Question #	Answer Here	Health Credit	Health Debit	Health Balance
1							1					
2							2					
3							3					
4							4					
5							5					
6							6					
7							7					
8							8					
9							9					
10							10					
11							11					
12							12					
13							13					
14							14					
15							15					
16							16					
17							17					
18							18					
19							19					
20							20					
21							21					
22							22					
23							23					
24							24					
25							25					
26							26					
27							27					
28							28					
28							29					
30							30					

Copy form for additional recording

HEALTHIOLOGY PLAYERS ACCOUNT SCORE CARD

Player: _____   Player: _____

Game #	Question #	Answer Here	Health Credit	Health Debit	Health Balance		Game #	Question #	Answer Here	Health Credit	Health Debit	Health Balance
1							1					
2							2					
3							3					
4							4					
5							5					
6							6					
7							7					
8							8					
9							9					
10							10					
11							11					
12							12					
13							13					
14							14					
15							15					
16							16					
17							17					
18							18					
19							19					
20							20					
21							21					
22							22					
23							23					
24							24					
25							25					
26							26					
27							27					
28							28					
28							29					
30							30					

Copy form for additional recording

Rate Yourself

18–20: Excellent   10–12:   Fair
15–17: Very Good   8–9:   Poor
13–14: Good   7 and Under: Fail, and needs urgent medical and health attention

NAME	Strongly Poor → Strongly Excellent						
	8	10	12	14	16	18	20
1							
2							
3							
4							

NAME	Strongly Poor → Strongly Excellent						
	8	10	12	14	16	18	20
1							
2							
3							
4							

NAME	Strongly Poor → Strongly Excellent						
	8	10	12	14	16	18	20
1							
2							
3							
4							

NAME	Strongly Poor → Strongly Excellent						
	8	10	12	14	16	18	20
1							
2							
3							
4							

★ ★ ★ ★ ★   ★ ★ ★ ★   ★ ★ ★   ★ ★   ★
EXCELLENT   VERY GOOD   GOOD   FAIR   POOR

Copy form for more player(s)

Rate Yourself

18–20: Excellent   10–12:   Fair
15–17: Very Good   8–9:   Poor
13–14: Good   7 and Under: Fail, and needs urgent medical and health attention

NAME	Strongly Poor → Strongly Excellent						
	8	10	12	14	16	18	20
1							
2							
3							
4							

NAME	Strongly Poor → Strongly Excellent						
	8	10	12	14	16	18	20
1							
2							
3							
4							

NAME	Strongly Poor → Strongly Excellent						
	8	10	12	14	16	18	20
1							
2							
3							
4							

NAME	Strongly Poor		Strongly Excellent					
	8	10	12	14	16	18	20
1								
2								
3								
4								

★ ★ ★ ★ ★   ★ ★ ★ ★   ★ ★ ★   ★ ★   ★

EXCELLENT   VERY GOOD   GOOD   FAIR   POOR

Copy form for more player(s)

Postscript

William Lucyk at 101

I once asked a friend's parents what the secret was to a happy marriage, since they were going on seventy-three years together, and still shared their heart and soul with one another as if they'd just met. Without hesitation William said, "There's no secret. Our marriage is an open book of how we live and have been able to maintain happiness throughout the years. Don't expect peace with your wife, if you aren't willing to compromise," said the husband. "Like everything else, there need to be insteps. It's one, two, three steps, and you have to be in harmony. It takes two people to work together. You can't expect one person to work at the harmony."

What I also learned from this 101-year-old William was something quite considerably important, something that most of us take for granted—our health. For decades, he and his wife spend time attending to their gardens, eating a well-balanced diet, reading and doing at least 30 minutes of exercise every day for their health.

Why health, nutrition and exercise is so important to this centurion? In the 60's after William developed ear problems, doctors told him there was nothing that they could do for him. They told him he should learn to live with it. However, nausea made him vomit at times and he had a loss of balance. William knew he had to do something about it, so he went to the library in Saskatoon, Canada and researched the first known nutritionist, Adele Davis. He bought the suggested powdered supplements in a Health Food Store. He drank this and got better. Since then he knew he had to be in charge of his own health and read many books on nutrition, and also practiced good health and daily exercises.

William's wife Lily, who turned ninety-seven-years old in March 2007, has been an avid gardener. They have always eaten from creation, planting their gardens with fruits, vegetables and herbs during the summer months. These two health conscious lovebirds who have been married for almost three quarters of a century still live in their own home, tend to the garden, fruit trees and picks pails of fruits to deliver to the neighbors and give away to passersby. The secret from William's and Lilly's lives that I took away is: We cannot take our health for granted. So the healthiest thing to do right now is to slowly break out of your bad eating habits, an hour or a day at a time. Soon good health is no longer a second place in your life, but first place.

Meanwhile, in the United States, weight loss remains a growing multi-billion-a-year business, with people looking for the 'perfect' diet pill that kept failing them, those in need for a 'quick fix', to loose the pounds. *Healthiology 101* is the game that was designed to help empower you to make choices. It was designed to help you change your thinking about your health. To use the information and take action on it, to stay focused, live healthy, and put an end to diet failure, by changing old habits and replace them with new ones, one day at a time.

You cannot starve yourself and expect to be healthy, and you cannot eat all you want and lose weight. That's only a perception. Even if you were to create a visualization about your health by using the starvation method or over-eating approach, it would not create a solid foundation for self-improvement, because you have handled your health the wrong way.

You must adhere to good diets, exercise and so forth; otherwise you could become another statistic. In one year alone, four hundred ninety-five thousand women in America lost their lives to cardio-vascular diseases. And we cannot forget nervosa, as millions of children and adults are living with this disease, because they are afraid of gaining weight. It is a serious, chronic and life-threatening disorder, and it too is out of control with children as young as five years old.

We are living longer than ever, but do you want to live in chronic pain, disease and misery, if you can avoid it? The *Healthiology 101* game will help you to reflect on your own health and others around you, like your children or spouse, and how to prevent some diseases from happening. The game is a lifestyle changing game to help you learn more about your own body and how you can prevent certain diseases from occurring or how to maintain whatever disease you already have so you can benefit from a better quality of the life that is left in you.

God created you in your own image, which is: You are not likely to fit into somebody else's mold, and neither anyone will fit into yours. So quit worrying yourself about the 'too thin' or 'too fat' hypocrisy of yourself, stop wanting to look like *somebody else*, and take charge of your life on how you plan to make yourself healthy.

It is never too late to take care of your health, but are you going to wait until something unhealthy happens? Do you plan to go down the unhealthy lifestyle ramp or cruise on the healthy lifestyle path? Do not wait to get ill or to come down with a preventive disease before you begin good health keeping. You can be like William. In the 60's, after he developed ear problems, doctors told him there was nothing that they could do for him. They told him he should learn to live with it. But he did not want to live and not able to hear. So he did something quite remarkable. He researched on nutrition, took a hold of his life and learned how take his health into his own hands. You can turn your health around from where you are, but the sooner the better. It is easier to get better health-wise when you start from early on.

Sometimes too much advice can be confusing. You have seen conflicting opinions about diets? There are thousands of diet books on the bookshelves, yet you hear they do not work. What you need to do is to use something as simple, yet so profound—use your imagination. Your imagination is extremely power-ful. You can use it to create positive or negative images of yourself. Negative thoughts bring out negative results. So when negative thoughts come in, cast them out immediately. Reprogram your negative thoughts and replace them with positive ones.

A thought is a reflection of your imagination. Your imagination is like a can-vas. The picture you paint is exactly the emotions of what you experienced on the inside is what comes out on the canvas. Until you can get a positive image of yourself, from the inside, you will never be able to paint a positive image or take care of yourself. So, stop debiting your health *account* and begin to credit your health by taking charge of it.

Our attitudes play an important role in our health. Talk is cheap. Do not cheap talk yourself out of good health. You should never allow your feelings to take control over your life. William did not! He reprogrammed himself to believe that he would hear again—that his hearing would get better. Almost half-a-century later he is still in control of his health at 101. As a result of his healthy actions, his wife Lilly and daughter Zora practices good health keeping skills. Since I met the family in 2004, I took a page out of their health methods, and am working on my own health too.

Take control of your health and place it into your own hands. Challenge your health and venture a bit further than you have gone before. How you see your health and how you feel about your health will have a tremendous impact on your overall health. I invite you to stand in front of a mirror. Do you see what I see? Is that the image you want to live with? What are you looking to change? Begin to accept yourself, right where you are, including the faults. Tell yourself that this is going to be the very minute you are going to take charge of your health. Paint a picture in your mind about your health and of what you want your health to be and conceive it from your heart. Believe it and begin to work on your health, because that is the only way you are going to do something about your health and work at it.

A train of thought about your health you should keep in mind is: The only place where 'success' comes before 'work' is in the dictionary. Health is not *one* thing. Health is not only about size. Therefore, to gain success with your health, you are going to need to first work at it by eating a well-balanced diet, exercise regularly, meditate, drink lots of water and get plenty of sleep; get regular medical check-ups—at least once a year, as part of our ongoing health lifestyle changes.

This generation could have less of a life expectancy than their parents and grandparents. So who will likely live a happier and healthier life? The persons who follow the health protocol or the persons who did nothing about their health? I think you know the answer. Regardless of medical advances and doctors, they cannot replace the individual's responsibility for every day good health practices. A doctor can help you to a certain degree, but you have to heal yourself by watching what you eat.

Reflection

Stress Healer

A lot of our well being is influenced by a great amount of stress in our daily lives. There is good stress and bad stress. However, what we are analyzing in this book is *bad stress*. We may think it is out of our control to alleviate the bad stress, but there are some things that can be done to be of help by getting rid of any obvious poor lifestyle habits and negative thoughts.

Stress and junk food make a fattening partnership, and certainly lead to other symptoms, illnesses and diseases. Everyone has a role to play in their health. My philosophy is: Confront life, be honest about your health, and then you may find that you have neglected yourself for all those years. Then you will be inspired to take charge of your health. In so doing, you will become an inspiration to others.

The primary role in *Healthiology 101* is to assist people in reaching their potential health goal. Stress plays a big role on our health. Have you ever stopped once in a while and ask yourself this question: *Am I healthy?* So why are you so worried if you a size 0 or a size 24 than about your general health? Most health problems begin with a six-letter word—stress. Worrying will only put extra stress on your mind. Stress is not only damaging your physical body, but also to your mind and spirit. It is much harder to lose weight if you are stressed or depressed. You can fix the stress, but you first need to focus on changing your lifestyle habits. Stress will steal away your joy.

Instead of wasting away precious time for unimportant things, take the time to start with inner peace by letting go of your stress; inhale a breath of fresh air and let it go into the bottom of your belly, exhale and tell yourself that you are getting rid of all the superfluity and overabundance of glut inside. Come on! You can do it. Exhale and begin to nourish and foster good things in your thoughts. To help you get there, start with things we often take for granted, like something as simple as sleep. Make sure you have enough sleep, because stress will drain all the energy out of your body.

Relaxation is one of the most effective self-help activities for stress on the body, mind and soul. Relaxation helps to clear your emotional climate. Tone down with a book or music to relax before going to bed. Here are some simple stress healers you should follow:

Take baths. An uninterrupted, romantic warm bath is like a tonic to rejuvenate your soul. It is like medicine. Fill your bathtub with soft water; add three tablespoonfuls of bubble bath and some bath salt; light your favorite candle; put on your most cherished CD; sink yourself in the bath and soak up with a soothing glass of your favorite drink. (Avoid alcohol as a de-stressor or any chemical anesthetic supplements.) Finish off with a light rinse and add some bath oil to complete your bath. This is a great refresher for a tired and stressful mind and body.

Read books. Books and literature are a holistic approach to relaxation. Pick a book or two of romance, suspense or a novel that you can hardly part with or want to put down. A book with humor is meritorious. Humor keeps us together to help lower our stress level, and a good book helps to get your mind away from the daily stresses. You can also purchase or borrow Books-on-CD from your local library.

Enjoy moderate exercise. Exercise can help you feel better, live longer and build strength. Regular exercise ensures that you stay mentally healthy, fit and strong. Do something that you like such as individual or group body exercises. Tai chi, yoga or walking; kickboxing and running are some of the different exercises that you can take to calm the nerves and stay focused. (See your doctor before you start exercising.)

A green house date adds flavor. A perfect environment for buds and blooms can decrease your stress. Slowly walk through the garden or plants making a connection with each one of them. Look at the flowers, touch them tenderly, smell their buds and blooms. Envision that they hold the secret to your heart and they are the truth to set you free from your stress. Flowers are the most romantic creation that sparkles your delight. Flowers are a paradise to fill an empty soul. They add a taste of beauty around you.

Meditation is a great stress reliever, and it does not take up a lot of energy in doing it. Meditation adds comfort to your soul and encompasses your ability to reach a state of serenity. With a soothing voice, specially created music and images create a wonderful experience. You can borrow a book from the library or purchase one that will help to still your mind, but first you must focus and still the mind to bring in the present—something that is good. Everyone is encouraged to meditate for a moment, and experience that peacefulness meditation brings to your soul. Begin to practice meditation for relaxing the body and calming the mind. First, find a quiet location where you can relax and focus undisturbed. It is a spiritual enlightenment for inner peace and natural balance. If you find negative thoughts entering your mind, stop what you are doing, do not give up, but refocus and start the meditation process again.

Music is a powerhouse. Soothing music is a welcome addition to meditation and healing. The sounds will enhance relaxation. So listen to the beat of the music, hum or sing along with it. Reach out for your partner and hold closely together for a dance or just to listen to each heartbeat and the sound of precious music. Or simply meditate on the words in the song to induce the mind to calm, to bring peace to the inner soul and relax the stressful body. Everyone has his or her personal preference of music, but softer or classical music adds a relaxing mode to a stressful mind, body and soul.

Nutrition is all about health. Health is the ultimate democracy of our body. Listen to your body, because it carries a story. We are what we eat. Watch your nutrition and eat healthy meals by adding quality fresh fruits, vegetables, whole-wheat grains, proteins, minerals, carbohydrates and use fat wisely. Increase your vitality and productivity through healthy eating and discover the importance to your well being that quality food groups can do for you and your body and how they can reduce stress.

People are the make-up of this great universe. Whether you know it or not, other people allow us to exist in the beautiful world of ours. We need people as long as we are alive, because we are not an island and we cannot exist on our own. Importantly, no one should have to be alone when they are experiencing any forms of stresses. No matter the situation there is always someone that you can get connected with. Develop and build a bond with people. It requires give-and-take of trust to make relationships work. Relationships do work. They have worked in the past, and relationships will continue to work now and in the future. To simply put it, we all need these emotional connections with other people; family, friends or co-workers to help us alleviate the stressors in our lives. Then we will be able to truly survive in the world.

Pets can be adorable little creatures or something as big as a horse. A pet is to be recommended during a stressful time. They improve the quality of people's personal and professional lives. Household pets provide spiritual qualities such as unconditional love, courage, joy, healing, patience, consistency, forgiveness and gratitude. Pets can add healthy and spiritual moments to human's stressful life.

Planet earth is all about health. Specifically, it is all about taking care of your health so that you can take care of the environment. Not taking care of your health, you are killing yourself and also harming the planet. What we eat affects the tone of our mind, body and soul, which gives off negative energies. Bad eating habits and negative energies process unhealthy waste-matters, which passes out of our bodies into the environment. We want to improve the environment, not to deface it. Our unhealthy habits are largely responsible for years of environmental abuses, as poorly waste-matters cannot give nourishment to purify the earth. Your health is the solution to planet earth. So you can only protect your health and the environment when you take care of *your* self, to truly enjoy and reap greatness in an immaculate environment on planet earth.

Sex is another stress reliever that people sometimes take for granted. Nothing beats good old sex for mature adults. Therefore, experience sexual extremities and enjoy an enduring intimacy with your partner. It helps to relieve your body and mind from stress and tensions. Romantic fantasies lessen pain and promote relaxation. Block the stress by fantasizing or recall romantic times spent with a special someone. It will help to expand your orgasms and produce sexual energy that will stimulate and heal you for hours after love-making.

Sleep is vital, like the breath you breathe to stay alive. It allows your body to relax and your brain to switch off so that the cells can rebuild and then start up refreshed, renewed and rejuvenated. Everyone needs sleep to build up your energy level to fight off sickness and combat stress. Life balance can reduce stress by making sure that you get the required amount of eight to nine hours of sleep each day. When you are off on weekends, sleep in, turn the alarm clock off and relax.

You are not just a service tool for your workplace, husband, wife or children. Breaking away from the stress is symbolic to find a spa where you can spoil *your* self. Explore your inner self and indulge in pampering for as little as an hour or for as long a day or two. A beautifying and therapeutic treatment will leave you feeling relaxed and beautiful.

Take a vacation. A break from your familiar surroundings can improve your life both at work and home. Take a break and go on a trip. As a simple get-a-way from turning up for work, marriage and children is important; so too is time out very important for a stressed mind. A weekend, a week, two weeks or a month away will help to ease your stress level and give you clearer thinking on problems that need to be resolved. You may be energized to confront them in a positive way. It will also have a positive effect on your health. If you are a lone-parent family, put your children in the care of a family member or someone you can trust, and go away even for a day or night, and explore your inner self.

Walking adds energy. Walk in a peaceful setting, looking at the natural resources like trees, wild flowers or architectural buildings, at art, people, pets, etc. and create freedom in your mind, body and spirit. Take a fifteen-minute or half an hour a day and take a walk to achieve your inner peace by letting go of your stress. Think that this moment is yours as you take your walk and that you are free and powerful and nothing can stop you now. It will give you the confidence and energy to move past the stress.

Water is purity. We are water-based creatures, so you should introduce lots of water into your life, like drinking, as your bodies need water to operate most favorably—a natural purification process to maximize health. Or for tranquility and awesome experience, sit by the lake on the water's edge, listen to the water-falls, and skip stones. Dip your toes in and slowly get your feet wet; close your eyes and invite peace of mind in. Listen to the waves, the wind, and the birds and imagine the beauty around. Listen to the surf break, take a deep breath of fresh air and just absorb all the calmness around you. Enjoy every moment of your peace and when you are ready to go, get up and kick some water in the air and smile at the drops falling back in the lake. Use your hands to scoop some up and pour it over your face; daydream that you are kissing the water to say thank you for a beautiful and stress-free time.

Yoga offers a significant benefit to reduce stress. It prepares the body for a higher state. By focusing on the mind and relaxing the body, it will help to produce a quiet and calm frame of mind. As you practice yoga and begin to experience this calm frame of mind, concentrate on inner peace to relax or to promote fitness, sleep and energize the body, mind and soul and bring them to freedom.

Learning these stress healers will definitely help you to relax and bring calmness to a stressful mind. Simply begin to slowly introduce each one of them into your daily lives. For instance, if you are meditating and if you find you are going back into your *old self*, stop whatever you are doing, refocus and think on the positive things you have recently created. Continue to focus and still your mind to bring your mind back to the present. Refocusing on positive things will help you get over the hurdles. The only route to a healthy lifestyle is to practice living it. Do not for a minute believe that practice makes *perfect*, but rather, believe without a shadow of a doubt that practice makes *improvement*. So practice, practice and do more practice to improve on your health.

As a society, we have to change the current trend of fast food and non-existence of exercise, to enable all of us to lead healthier lives, without sacrificing the generation of *tomorrow*. Everyone needs time and fun to relax. Use Healthiology book or board game to help you relax and calm your stress. This game not only helps us to develop healthy lifestyles, but also allow us to have fun while playing it. Moreover, when we get together in groups to play the *Healthiology 101* game, it will add pleasurable fun, excitement and knowledge to our inquisitive minds. Then we will take further interest to find out more about our bodies and what we could do to improve upon it.

Finally, families must learn to be inclusive, to share, as it is by sharing that you can learn about others and yourself. Good luck with your health, and the health of your loved ones.

FIND A WORD THE HEALTY WAY WITH HEALTHIOLOGY

O	R	A	N	G	E	S	C	B	M	W	M	I	L	H
T	A	S	P	I	N	B	H	R	U	A	C	W	C	O
O	C	A	B	B	A	G	E	O	S	G	D	A	A	R
M	A	L	P	A	P	R	D	C	H	N	N	T	B	S
A	R	M	A	P	P	A	F	I	R	I	R	E	G	E
I	M	O	C	P	L	E	B	J	P	K	V	R	N	R
H	U	N	O	C	H	E	E	S	E	L	J	U	M	A
U	S	S	P	I	N	S	S	A	L	A	L	N	S	D
C	H	I	C	K	E	N	B	A	J	W	E	H	T	I
J	R	S	L	E	E	B	R	O	U	M	E	U	O	S
O	O	U	H	U	M	R	R	U	M	C	O	M	R	H
G	O	N	O	N	I	O	N	S	P	R	E	O	R	M
G	M	N	R	R	M	C	S	L	P	A	X	Z	A	I
I	S	I	S	U	Y	C	J	S	L	E	E	P	C	L
N	F	C	H	I	C	O	S	S	C	O	R	X	I	O
G	R	R	L	F	H	L	I	N	R	A	C	Y	L	R
T	O	M	E	I	E	I	F	I	S	M	I	L	K	U
L	E	E	K	S	E	S	M	S	J	U	S	T	B	N
I	C	A	S	H	J	O	G	I	E	X	E	R	E	N
M	O	U	B	E	A	R	A	O	R	A	N	G	A	I
G	R	A	P	E	S	U	R	R	U	N	N	I	N	G
B	N	W	A	L	K	T	O	M	A	T	O	E	S	S

Applesauce	Chicken	Jogging	Running
Beans	Corn	Jump	Salmon
Broccoli	Exercise	Leeks	Sleep
Brussels sprout	Fish	Milk	Spinach
Cabbage	Grapes	Mushrooms	Tomatoes
Carrots	Horse Radish	Oranges	Walking
Cheese	Humor	Raisins	Water

Healthiology Definition

Definition: *Healthiology* is the art of good health practices; the theory and practice of personal and individual health keeping; it deals with the application of daily health practices in the areas of a well-balanced diet, daily exercise, meditation and regular medical check-ups.

* * * * *

Our health and well being is of utmost importance. Living healthy and knowing that our children are healthy too, takes knowledge and nourishing lifestyle practices. *Healthiology 101* not only helps us to develop these lifestyles, but also allow us to have fun while doing so with preventative measures.

We have one life to live, so while we develop these healthy practices for ourselves, let us bear in mind that we also have a generation to care for. Let us start with the children, as we seek to create a healthy generation, starting with baby steps today.

* * * * *

Look for *Common Sense for Young Minds, Healthiology: Pangella, the Health Nerd and Friends* DVD and coloring book that are part of the children's healthy growing up series.

How to Purchase a Book Without the Board Game

The *Healthiology 101* hbk, pbk and ebk can be purchased individually, from the publisher, iUniverse at 1-800-288-4677; online stores at: **www.iuniverse.com**, **www.barnesandnoble.com**, **www.amazon.com** or from **bookstores**.

P.S. The board game can be purchased at **www.healthiology.com**

Healthiology Certificate

The Healthiology certificate belongs to you, *the player(s)*, after you have read, completed the quiz book or board game task, and followed the excellent health practices in your personal health keeping.

HEALTHIOLOGY
The Active Body Culture Game

Presents this

Certificate of Unmasked Health

To

_____

(Fill in your name upon completion of the game rules)

Having successfully participated in the Healthiology quiz and/or board game; and in recognition for effectively following the rules about good health practices in the areas of a well-balanced diet, daily exercise, meditation and regular medical check-ups, and in Witness Whereof my signature is hereto affixed

This _____ day of _____ 2 _____

(Fill in the month, date and year upon completion of the game rules)

_____
MWilson
M. M. Wilson, Author

You can make copies of the certificate for other players who have followed the game rules.

About the Author

M. M. Wilson's books have been described as 'life changing' *BREAD, MILK AND LOVE HAVE EXPIRATION DATES* give us true stories of peoples experience with love; *MURDER BY DECEPTION IN PARIS*' encourages travelers to be more aware of their surroundings when they visit foreign countries, while *COMMON SENSE FOR YOUNG MINDS* is a life-changing parent and child relationship development book. Wilson lives in Mississauga, Ontario, Canada.

Available for Christmas!

FUN IN THE KITCHEN:
The Cookbook for Men

978-0-595-47103-4
0-595-47103-X